HEALTH CARE WITHOUT WALLS: A ROADMAP FOR REINVENTING U.S. HEALTH CARE

Susan Dentzer, Editor

CONTENTS

ACKNOWLEDGMENTS 3
INTRODUCTION: Why Create a Future of Health Care Without Walls? 5
Health Care Without Walls: Introductory Chapter in Brief................................... 21
Scenario 1: A Man Seeking State-of-the-Art Cancer Care in a Remote Setting....24
Scenario 2: An Elderly Woman, Living Alone, With Mild Cognitive Impairment and Chronic Conditions.. 27
Chapter 1: Technology and Health Care Without Walls 31
Scenario 3: A Teen With Diabetes and Father With Congestive Heart Failure Stay at Home with Their Conditions Controlled.. 73
Scenario 4: A Chronically Ill Couple in a Rural Area 77
Chapter 2: Payment and Reimbursement to Support Health Care Without Walls 81
Scenario 5: A Young Boy with Developmental and Physical Disabilities 125
Chapter 3: Regulatory Changes to Support Health Care Without Walls.............. 128
Scenario 6: A Woman Recovering from Breast Cancer 160
Chapter 4: The Work Force to Support Health Care Without Walls 162
Scenario 7: A Pregnant Woman At High Risk for Pregnancy Complications and Premature Birth 222
Chapter 5: Human Factors in Designing Heath Care Without Walls................... 226
Scenario 8: Virtual Care and Pandemic Influenza.. 257

ACKNOWLEDGMENTS

THIS REPORT was produced under the auspices of the Health Care Without Walls initiative, a program of the Network for Excellence in Health Innovation (NEHI). NEHI is a nonprofit, nonpartisan organization with nearly 100 members across all key sectors of health care. NEHI's mission is to advance innovations that improve health, enhance the quality of health care, and achieve greater value for the money spent. NEHI convenes and consults with its membership, and conducts independent, objective research and convenings, to accelerate these innovations and bring about changes within health care and in public policy.

The Health Care Without Walls initiative would not have been possible without the generous support of a number of several organizations: the Gordon and Betty Moore Foundation; the Jewish Healthcare Foundation (JHF); the California Healthcare Foundation (CHCF); Sanofi; the Inova health system; and Advanced ICU Care. We especially thank Julie Lawrence of the Moore Foundation; Karen Wolk Feinstein of the JHF; Barbara N. Lubash, Board Member Emerita of CHCF; Amit Rastogi, MD, of Inova; and Andrea Clegg of Advanced ICU Care for their enthusiastic support of the project. The program was carried out by five work streams, focused on technology, payment and reimbursement, regulatory issues, the health care work force, and human factors issues.

The leadership teams of all five work streams were as follows:

- **Technology**: Barbara DeBuono, MD, MPH, Vice President, Clinical Strategy and Value Based Care, 3M Health Information Systems; Karen Murphy, PhD, RN, Chief Innovation Officer, Geisinger Health System; Amit Rastogi, MD, MHCM, Senior Vice President for Strategy, Growth and Innovation, Inova Health System; Sara Vaezy, MHA, MPH, Chief Digital Strategy Officer,

Providence St. Joseph Health; and Joel Vengco, MS, MA, Chief Information Officer/Senior Vice President, Baystate Health

- **Payment and Reimbursement**: John Bulger, DO, MBA, Chief Medical Officer, Geisinger Health Plan; Mark Lutes, JD, MA, Chair, Board of Directors, Epstein Becker Green; Severence MacLaughlin, Global Head for Artificial Intelligence and Data Sciences in Healthcare & Life Sciences, and Head, Artificial Intelligence Learning Institute and Cognizant Academy of Data Sciences, Cognizant Technology Solutions; Sunny Ramchandani, MD, MPH, Deputy Chief Medical Officer, Aetna; and Karen Rheuban, MD, Director, University of Virginia Center for Telehealth

- **Regulatory Issues:** James Boiani, JD, Member of the Firm, Epstein Becker Green, and Andrea Clegg, MBA, Chief Financial Officer, Advanced ICU Care.

- **Work Force:** Julene Campion, MS, SPHR, SPC, Vice President, Talent Acquisition, Geisinger Health System; Anita McDonnell, RPh, Former Vice President, Government Health Initiatives and Political Action, Sanofi; and Carla Smith, MA, CNM, FHIMSS, Executive Vice President, HIMSS

- **Human Factors:** Pascale Carayon, PhD, Procter and Gamble Bascom Professor in Total Quality/Director of the Center for Quality and Productivity Improvement, University of Wisconsin-Madison; Frances Dare, MBA, Managing Director, Health Strategy Practice, Accenture; Dan Gillette, EdM, Principal Investigator, Public Health Institute; Sr. Research Scientist and Co-Director of Tech for Social Good, CITRIS, University of California at Berkeley.

Several writers also assisted in preparation of draft chapters of this report, as follows: Joan Stephenson, Steven Findlay, Charles Babington, Helaine Resnick, and Erin Hammers Forstag. I thank them for their diligent and thoughtful work. Finally, members of the NEHI team worked tirelessly to support the Health Care Without Walls initiative and the execution on this report: Valerie Fleishman, Lauren Choi, Tim Tassa, Yaminah Romulus, Sanja Mutabdzija, Tom Hubbard, Pamela Milton, Amanda Mehlman, and Margo Perez. I thank them, most of all, for being marvelous colleagues, dedicated to the work of improving health and health care.

Susan Dentzer, Editor
President and Chief Executive Officer, NEHI (the Network for Excellence in Health Innovation)
Washington, DC, October 2018

INTRODUCTION: WHY CREATE A FUTURE OF HEALTH CARE WITHOUT WALLS?

IMAGINE A health care system that came to people, meeting them where they are, in their homes, workplaces, or elsewhere in their communities—rather than expecting people to always go to it.

Imagine a system that anticipated individuals' needs, worked to keep them as healthy as possible, and viewed any need to access "sick care" as letting them down.

Imagine a system that was as convenient and accessible as other elements of life that people now take for granted, such as sending money with an app on a mobile phone, or ordering groceries online.

That system could be called Health Care Without Walls.

Now imagine the people who, despite their health challenges, might thrive in such a system:

- An elderly woman with mild cognitive impairment. Instead of moving into assisted living, or to a nursing home, she could remain in her own home—while both her health care providers and adult daughter kept tabs on her through remote monitoring systems.

- A single mother with a physically and developmentally disabled child confined to a wheelchair. Instead of struggling with transportation to get her child to various medical appointments, she could meet by video with the care team to help plan the child's care.

- A couple with multiple chronic illnesses, who live in a rural area with few health care options. They could have telehealth visits with specialists at distant academic medical center—including psychotherapy for the husband's depression, and wellness coaching to help the wife with her self-care for diabetes.

- A city full of people frightened by an outbreak of pandemic influenza. People with flu symptoms could take self-administered tests for the flu virus, and if they tested positive, could have antiviral medicine delivered to their doorsteps. Mass online public health "clinics" would urge healthy people to stay at home until the epidemic ebbed.

What if more care could be delivered virtually to patients such as these, outside of the conventional physical settings of hospitals and physicians' offices? Although not automatically an unmitigated upside, a move to more virtual, "distributed" care delivery outside of the conventional physical settings would have many advantages. These benefits could include greater access to care for the many people who live in underserved areas of the United States, and the world; increasing convenience for consumers; removing some of the "friction" in health care, or the components that add to time, work, and expense, without directly producing more health or better care; and potentially lowering the cost of care.

NEHI, the Network for Excellence in Health Innovation, has just such a vision for health care in 2025: that it will be increasingly accessed and delivered "without walls." With the benefit of technologies such as telehealth, patients will receive more care than they do now in their homes, schools, and other community-based venues and "distributed" settings out of conventional health care settings, such as hospitals and physicians' offices. Care will be delivered by multidisciplinary teams of providers, who will combine their clinical competencies with technology and informatics in patient care. Focused more on people in their communities—where they live, learn, work, and play—these multidisciplinary teams will also address the social and economic determinants of health that often drive illness and care needs.

Of course, not all of health care could or should be "delivered" to individuals' homes or work sites. If you were in a bad car accident, you'd still want to be taken to the nearest high-level trauma center for treatment—and if you think you're having a heart attack, to a hospital emergency department, right away.

But many aspects of health care do not involve the same or similar degree of "laying on of hands" that would be needed in these dire circumstances. They are more about exchanges of information: Of a patient relaying symptoms to a doctor, or of a doctor reading the results of tests and consulting with a patient about next steps.

In almost all other aspects of modern life, most people are becoming accustomed to exchanging information like this by phone, or over the Internet—in other words, virtually. In health care—perhaps more than in almost any other aspect of contemporary life—the default standard in much of the country is still to exchange such information in person—physically, in an office, clinic, or emergency department visit. And notwithstanding the advent of electronic health records, and patient portals into them, huge volumes of health care information are exchanged daily over telephone lines by facsimile machine, or fax, a technology first introduced in the 1960s. The antiquated nature of these processes is one reason that wags have joked that the U.S. health care system delivers "Star Wars" medicine on a "Flintstones" delivery platform.

But thanks to the advent of technologies, including information technology and the digitization of health care data, health care is already changing. As the science fiction writer William Gibson once remarked, "The future is already here—it's just not very evenly distributed." Consider these examples of the "future" that are already in place:

- Within the Kaiser Permanente Health system—which now boasts 12.2 million enrollees across 8 states and the District of Columbia—more than 50 percent of the roughly 120 million "visits" annually now take place over the phone, email, or video.

- At the University of Virginia health system, based in Charlottesville, VA, telemedicine programs across multiple specialties—ranging from dermatology and wound care to genetic counseling and high-risk pregnancy support—have been estimated to save patients more than 17 million miles of driving over roughly the past decade.

- In New York City, people can walk into a Walgreens or Duane Reade pharmacy and, from a kiosk, have a video visit with an emergency physician at Weill Cornell Medical/New York Presbyterian Health system. At least once in 2018, a middle-aged man suffering from multiple chronic conditions who appeared to be on the verge of a heart attack was able to be diagnosed quickly via this service, and was transported to a hospital for immediate care.

- Outside the United States, innovation in "health care without walls" approaches if anything is even more advanced. In parts of England, patients in the National health Service can choose "GP in Hand," a mobile consultation service powered by artificial intelligence, to check their symptoms on a mobile app and, if needed, book a virtual visit with a physician thereafter.[1] In Norway, a partnership between the Norwegian telecommunications company Telenor and the health system aims to have one-third of the country's kidney failure patients to undergo dialysis at home, with the aid of a digital tool to send information directly to hospitals for monitoring purposes.[2]

- Meanwhile, in Bangladesh, 5 million subscribers to the Grameenphone cellular phone service have signed up for Tonic—a unique combination of an app, insurance coverage, and telehealth service rolled into one. For the equivalent of just 60 cents per month, Tonic subscribers get $500 in hospital coverage; 10 minutes a month of consultations with physicians by phone, 24/7; discounts on medications and health services—all with the goal of providing the largely uninsured Bangladeshi population with "world-class healthcare."[3]

- Not all examples of "Health Care Without Walls" involve technologies such as apps or telehealth. At Wake Forest Baptist medical center in North Carolina, eight community health workers, dubbed "supporters of health," work with formerly hospitalized patients to enable them to stay at home and avoid readmissions to the hospital. They visit patients in their home, and assist with coordinating primary care visits, providing transportation to their medical appointments, arranging access to medications and food, and connecting them with other needed services available in the community.[4,5]

As we at NEHI contemplated these examples and imagined other possibilities, we began to think about other types of individuals who could benefit from a more distributed health care system, and the many obstacles in their path. We began to imagine someone named Dave.

Imagining the Possibilities: The Fictional Story of Dave

In our mind's eye, Dave is a man in his 40s, living on Kodiak Island, Alaska. He's a natural scientist with a PhD; is healthy and active; and spends a good deal of time outdoors, hiking and fishing.

One day Dave develops a hacking cough, which persists for several weeks, and then to more than month. After postponing a trip to the doctor, he eventually decides to be seen, and makes his way to the critical access hospital on Kodiak Island, to consult with the primary care physicians, and possibly other specialists, there.

The physician who sees him is concerned about the duration of the cough, and performs a full workup, including a chest x-ray. A suspicious x-ray leads to an MRI. The doctor tells Dave he's got a mass in his lung, and suspects lung cancer.

Dave is devastated, but as a scientist, his natural inclination is to spring into action and conduct research. While he awaits further tests, he goes home, and gets on the Internet.

Within hours, Dave, a healthy nonsmoker, has already read the equivalent of volumes about lung cancer. He determines that, if he does have lung cancer, it's most likely that he has non-small-cell lung cancer, which is frequently associated with nonsmoking. He reads about sophisticated targeted cancer therapies that have been developed to treat it, and that extend life considerably in some sufferers. He finds out that much of the groundbreaking research and treatment for this condition is taking place at major cancer centers, such as in New York, or Houston. He learns that, to get the optimal treatment, he should have his cancer's genome decoded, and his own genome as well.

At this point, Dave reflects on his options. Take a leave of absence from his job, and fly to a city such as New York or Houston for further consultation and treatment? Take up residence in either city for an indefinite time? He has good health insurance, but not unlimited financial resources to put himself up in a hotel for a long stay. How will he swing a potentially costly and prolonged episode of care?

Then Dave, as a scientist and a patient, decides that he has better ideas. In this modern day and age, he should be able to have his test results sent to a premier oncologist on staff at a major cancer center. He should be able to have a telehealth consult with the oncologist to hear about his treatment options. The specialist will interpret Dave's genomic test results, he or she may even consult with a "cognitive computing" platform powered by analytics and artificial intelligence to arrive at the appropriate treatment plan. If the plan calls for a targeted therapy, the doctor should be able to e-prescribe it through a specialty pharmacy, and it should be sent to the hospital on Providence Island for the local staff to administer it to Dave. Perhaps the targeted therapy can even be delivered to the island by drone.

Dave expects health care to operate without walls, and with good reason. Everything he proposes to be done, could be done, technically. He could have his test results sent to faraway specialists, and could have a video "visit" with them via telehealth; they could arrive at a treatment plan, e-prescribe the targeted therapy, and it could be delivered to Kodiak Island. The only catch: As there isn't now regular drone service to Kodiak, they'll have to use an express delivery service, like FedEx, instead.

Although technically possible today, would any of this happen? Not on your life—or Dave's, either.

The first barrier to Health Care Without Walls is that the health care "system" just isn't set up to operate this way—to match patients to optimal treatment, and attempt to get it to them no matter where they are. The different clinicians and health care sites that would need to collaborate on Dave's care don't have an existing way to divide up the work load, or share any payments forthcoming from Dave's health insurer. The New York or Texas oncologist initially in charge of diagnosing and recommending treatment for Dave would need to get a license to practice medicine in Alaska to have a telehealth visit with him. There is no existing program to train the clinicians on Kodiak to treat Dave with the targeted therapy, or manage any side effects as they would be at the major cancer center.

Anyone in Dave's situation would want what he wants—to stay at home, and yet receive the best care available anywhere. Technically, it's all feasible. Realistically, today, it would never happen. In all likelihood, Dave would have to decamp from Kodiak Island and seek his treatment very far from home. The system would not bend to meet him and his needs; he would bend to meet the system. That's why there is a need for Health Care Without Walls.

Why Health Care Without Walls Must Happen

We at NEHI believe that it's a national imperative to move more toward a system of Health Care Without Walls, to capture the benefits cited above. And there are multiple trends under way in U.S. health care, in the economy, and in society, that make a system of Health Care Without Walls more achievable and necessary than ever.

On the positive side, information technology has advanced to such a degree that even the U.S. health care system—long a laggard in adopting such technology—is at last reaping the fruits of major investments in digitizing health care information. As discussed in the chapters that follow, the combination of digitized data, analytics, and various forms of so-called machine learning and artificial intelligence, is transforming the use of data and information in health care.

To state fact this is not to argue that all aspects of information technology in health care are positive, or that the digital transformation of care has been completed; as Robert Wachter, MD, author of *The Digital Doctor,* has noted, multiple harms and unanticipated consequences also have occurred with "the dawn of medicine's computer age."[6] Yet it is also true that more data and information than ever are available to clinicians and others to understand what is happening with an individual patient, with populations of patients, and within the health care system overall. The fact that human beings have not yet fully determined how best to harness that information, or make it useful to clinicians, means only that there is far more work to be done.

An equally positive and related trend is the advent of precision medicine—the field that has yielded the targeted cancer therapies from which our fictional character, Dave, hopes to benefit, and that arguably constitutes the "Star Wars" aspects of modern medicine alluded to earlier. Francis Collins, director of the National Institutes of Health, has explained the development this way:

> **"For most of medicine's history, and with notable exceptions like blood transfusion, physicians have been forced to approach prevention and treatment of disease based on the expected response of an average patient because that was the best that could be done. However, a more precise, personalized approach to medicine is becoming possible. One major reason is that the cost of sequencing a human genome has declined substantially and is approaching $1,000—an astounding figure considering that it cost about $400 million to produce the first sequence of the human genome a little more than a decade ago."[7]**

Collins wrote those words in 2015. Three years later, in 2018, the cost of whole genome sequencing has dropped to about $600, and some commercial entities are aiming to bring the cost as low as $100 within several years.[8]

Cancer treatment is in the vanguard of the evolution of precision medicine, as growing understanding of the particular genomic and molecular drivers of different cancers has yielded an explosion of therapies aimed at these specific drivers. The same dynamics—multiple genomic and molecular drivers of the same underlying condition—may well apply to other disease states, such as diabetes.

The scientific drive to uncover such truths is one of the motivators of the "All of Us" trial[9] now under way under the auspices of NIH. The goal is to create a "research community" of 1 million people whose health information can be tracked over time, in part to identify risk factors for more diseases and assist in development of new treatments. After an initial visit to donate samples, such as of blood, urine, and to take physical measurements, participants will generally track and share their data remotely, on smart phones, and other devices with the aid of apps.

Clearly, technology and precision medicine are converging to create entirely new possibilities for advancing research, treatment, and human health. It's possible to conceive of new types of clinical trials, in which individuals with diabetes are wearing continuous glucose monitors powered by smart systems that automatically adjust their insulin levels to their desired targets. The same technologies can simultaneously collect and send information back to patients' clinicians, but also to researchers, who can study effects over time and parlay their knowledge back into ever more precise and sophisticated treatment.

Much of what's described above can occur without patients, researchers, and clinicians ever being in the same room together, unless they wish to do so. These exchanges could take place across miles, regions, even continents.

This, too, can be Health Care Without Walls.

A third trend that is positive for Health Care Without Walls, if potentially disruptive to other features of the health care landscape, is that care is already moving out of institutions such as inpatient hospitals, partly because technological change enables it, and partly because of convenience. Inpatient hospital admissions have been declining for years,[10] even as standalone surgery centers and emergency rooms, as well as urgent care centers, have proliferated. The volume of care delivered through retail clinics and urgent-care centers is also growing.

To be sure, some of these trends have had negative consequences for hospital finances. What's more, a number of studies have shown that care distributed in distributed settings or modes—whether retail clinics or telehealth—has led to more care being provided, and therefore to greater spending.[11] What isn't known is whether this increased care is superfluous, or whether these more convenient settings are addressing previously unmet needs. On the other hand, some analyses have shown lower costs from discrete telehealth services that could in theory produce savings, provided that they were not offset with a greater volume of services. A year-long Humana study (non-peer-reviewed, and as yet unpublished) of pairs of patients closely matched for diagnosis and other features showed that telemedicine visits were paid out at an average of $38 versus $114 for a face-to-face consultation.[12]

There are negative trends under way in U.S. health care that arguably compel creation of new systems of Health Care Without Walls.

First, U.S. health expenditure growth continues to outstrip the rate of growth of the economy,[13] and prices for nearly all health care goods and services in the nation exceed those paid for comparable services in other advanced nations.[14] In particular, the growth of the large and rising share of public spending devoted to health care is widely viewed as unsustainable. And with insurance premiums rising, and consumers' cost-sharing growing in absolute terms, much of health care is increasingly unaffordable to patients. These out-of-pocket costs come on top of the reality that wage and salary growth has undoubtedly been suppressed as more of overall compensation goes to pay for health care benefits.[15]

Second, by many measures, the level of health of much of the U.S. population is overall mediocre at best,[16] and is worsening for elements of the population, whose life expectancy has either declined or stopped increasing. Overall, U.S. life expectancy at birth is already below that of most other high-income countries, and is projected by 2030 to be similar to that of the Czech Republic for men, and Croatia and Mexico for women.[17]

The suboptimal state of social and economic determinants of health, such as incomes and education, offer one explanation, as do developments such as drug overdose deaths stemming from the opioid epidemic.[18] The trillions of dollars expended on health care are not reversing these overall grim trends.

The social and economic drivers of poor health, such as incomes and education, and the behaviors that often accompany them—overeating, lack of physical activity, or even substance abuse—take root and exist in communities, outside of the health care system.[19] Yet the health care system is where we devote most of our time and resources to addressing the ill effects. Many diseases are increasingly understood as the result of an interplay of genomics and other biological features, and the environment—where we live, what we eat, what we are exposed to.[20] Health care too frequently ignores about half of the equation—the environment in which people live their lives—until it is almost too late.

The Benefits of Health Care Without Walls

There is no guarantee that moving to a system of "Health Care Without Walls," propelled forward by the positive trends described above, would counteract these negative trends. But there is considerable potential that it could.

Convenience

As the chapters that follow lay out, Health Care Without Walls could drastically increase the convenience of care, meeting patients where they are—at home, at work, or elsewhere in the community. Already, parents and other caregivers of young children can use smart phone otoscope attachments to snap pictures of the inside of their children's' ears and transmit them to pediatric care providers, avoiding a trip to the doctor for suspected ear infections (although there is debate over whether images captured by parents and other nonprofessionals are suitable for diagnostic purposes[21,22]). Similarly, it's possible to imagine the use of multiple combinations of smart devices and telehealth applications across scores of conditions. Even if most patients or consumers aren't routinely using telehealth today, they appear to be increasingly open to trying it. A 2018 Deloitte survey showed that, although 77 percent of respondents had never tried a virtual visit, more than half (57 percent) were willing to do so.[23]

Health Care Without Walls could also leverage and extend the nation's corps of clinicians, providing far more care to the nation's thousands of underserved areas (officially labeled Health Professions Shortage Areas or Medically Underserved Areas, along with other designations). Consider: Entire counties of California lack any resident practicing psychiatrists whatsoever. But Mental health care needs can now be addressed through telepsychiatry services from health systems such as Sutter Health.[24]

Similarly, Health Care Without Walls could "democratize" and universalize clinical knowledge and expertise. Think of our fictional Dave having access to state-of-the art cancer care via his desired telehealth "visits" from Kodiak Island with far-off specialists. In the Internet age, when patients anywhere can read about state-of-the art medical breakthroughs and new protocols being used anywhere in the world, why should they or their clinicians not have access to the knowledge inherent in these advances?

Health Care Without Walls could help to reduce the unnecessary "friction" in system. Every day, there is lost productivity, and absenteeism, as people take time off from work or their other activities to transport themselves to health care sites, where they often sit and wait. There is huge "sunk" capital investment in large hospital buildings and other physical facilities that may not actually need to exist. Vast amounts of money, and human investment, goes into health care that arguably does not produce one real iota of additional health. It is not clear how much Health Care Without Walls would reduce this friction, but it is highly probable that it would do so to at least some degree.

It is axiomatic that most people do not spend most of their lives in the health care system, but rather in living in the community, where their social and economic circumstances strongly influence their health.[25] Even if they become ill and need health care, many people struggle to meet basic needs, such as for food, affordable and safe housing, and transportation. Health systems increasingly understand that they must partner with other community-based organizations to address these needs, lest people end up even sicker. In short, health systems already have to act beyond their walls and transcend conventional boundaries around health care. Systems of Health Care Without Walls would only reinforce and extend what the most enlightened health systems—such as Kaiser Permanente, Dignity Health, ProMedica, and others—are doing anyway.

Public health

Health Care Without Walls also constitutes an important opportunity to integrate both health care and public health. In the United States, the public health system is thought of, and mostly is, distinct from the health care system. This bifurcation is in contrast to other countries, where public health and medical care services are embedded in a centralized health system and social and health care policies are more integrated than they are in the United States.[26] But as U.S. health care "bridges" beyond its walls into the community, it has new opportunities to engage in, and complement, the health prevention and promotion activities that lie at the heart of public health: vaccinating children and adults to prevent the spread of disease; educating people about the risks of alcohol and tobacco; tracking and responding to diseases and epidemics; preventing injuries, and much more. Even if the health care and public health care systems will never be officially joined and centralized in the United States, each has the opportunity in a Health Care Without Walls environment to become a much more effective partner to the other.

Costs

There is no guarantee that Health Care Without Walls would be less expensive than the current system, even if friction is reduced, social needs are met, and much costly health care averted. For a host of reasons—including because a more distributed system may address health care needs that now go unmet—it is possible that spending would rise.

However, as discussed at length in the Payment and Reimbursement chapter of this volume, it is also possible that judicious payment systems could be devised that would lead less expensive forms of virtual care to supplant more costly care. And already there are examples of systems that can show that they've reduced total costs of care by moving to more virtual care delivery.

For example, in 2017, the Ascension Health system created the "Good Health Solutions Center," based in Texas, to create a seamless experience for patients by integrating scheduling across all of Ascension's local inpatient and outpatient care sites, care navigation, and virtual care services. In particular, the model provided new alternatives for telemedicine consultations between patients and clinicians. These virtual consultations, combined with on-demand access to care teams, produced dramatic results for heart failure patients recently discharged from hospitals. In just under a year, a group of these patients who received remote monitoring and virtual consultations had readmission rates of just 2.47 percent, versus 26 percent for a comparison group. Although these data have not yet been published and the results are still early, Ascension says that it appears as though high-risk patients who receive these technology-enabled care management services after hospital discharge have better outcomes, leading to better health and a substantial decrease in total costs of care.[27]

Barriers

As noted above, for all of the benefits that might accrue from a more distributed system of health care, multiple obstacles also stand in the way of it. There is a fundamental inertia in the health care system that has long proved resistance to disruptions created by new technology. Payment structures and regulations designed for older systems of care delivery, based on fee-for-service payment and physical visits to facilities such as hospitals, haven't proved to be readily adaptable to new delivery models. Today's health care work force isn't currently educated, trained, or equipped to deliver more technology-driven care in the age of Precision Medicine. And human factors that bear on how providers and patients will adapt to new modes of health care delivery are only partly understood.

As NEHI contemplated these realities, the goal of its Health Care Without Walls initiative became not only to frame a vision of a more distributed care system in 2025, but also to delineate the obstacles that stand in the way of this vision. Five "work streams" were formed to explore the possibilities of more technology-enabled care, along with the obstacles posed by payment and reimbursement, federal and state regulatory issues, the health care work force, and human factors. Based on careful examinations of anticipated barriers and opportunities, each work stream crafted recommendations for policy makers and other stakeholders that aim to expedite the transition to a more technology-enabled, distributed care delivery system. The work stream analyses also focused on knowledge gaps—the many things we still don't know about virtual care delivery, for example—and highlighted areas where additional work would need to be done to determine the impact on safety of care, quality of care, and costs.

The findings of the work streams are examined in detail in the chapters that follow. In brief, the work streams concluded that the state of technology is not at all the limiting factor in moving to a more distributed system, since dozens of technologies that could be put to constructive use in health care are already on the market. The barriers to a more distributed system lie elsewhere.

Aspects of **payment and reimbursement** of health care services are now being modified gradually to accommodate technologies such as telehealth, and to encourage new care models that focus more on social services and supports for patients. But still more new payment models are needed to support the adoption of technology, while displacing older forms of care that are likely to be duplicative, costlier and more inefficient to provide, or less useful or needed over time.

Multiple **regulatory** issues that must be grappled with are spread across broad categories, ranging from data privacy and security to governance of the Internet. These issues exist in today's health care system, to be sure, but they only become more acute in an environment when care is more distributed. As an example, it will be impossible to conduct robust systems of telehealth to reach America's most underserved communities without universal, affordable broadband Internet service.

The **work force** in health care most likely faces major upheavals, as jobs change, tasks performed by different types of workers change, and new skills and capabilities are needed. Current health care work force projections, such as for physicians, do not take technological changes into account, which means that the nation is in some sense flying blind about the types of workers who will be needed. Training and education of the health care work force will need to undergo major changes to prepare workers for a future of far more distributed, virtual care.

With respect to **human factors,** health systems, patients, and others must engage with technology developers to ensure the usability of technologies for diverse types of patients. The fact that today's voice assistants, such as Alexa and Siri, can't readily recognize English spoken with slight foreign accents[28] could prove harmful if such technologies were used in patient care, without these flaws being identified ahead of time, and fixed.

All of these challenges should be systematically addressed as best as possible to achieve the likely benefits of a more distributed delivery system. We at NEHI believe that these benefits will be real, and will bring enormous value to patients.

As NEHI's work streams conducted their analyses, in fact, they sought to keep individuals, patients, and families at the center of the Health Care Without Walls vision. A number of scenarios of hypothetical patients, along the lines of the story of Dave and the brief vignettes above, are spread throughout this volume. The scenarios help to paint a vivid picture of how aspects of the current health care system fail patients—and how a technology-enabled, more distributed system of prevention and care could serve them far better.

We hope that, before long, these hypothetical examples will be replaced by real-life examples of the people who will experience Health Care Without Walls—and of the dedicated clinicians and other members of the public health, health care, and social services systems who will serve them. As the old saying goes, the best way to predict the future is to create it—starting now.

◆ ◆ ◆

End Notes, Introduction

[1] Eric Wicklund, "Doctors' Protests Plague UK's Direct-to-Consumer Telehealth Service," mHealthIntelligence, April 04, 2018, https://mhealthintelligence.com/news/doctors-protests-plague-uks-direct-to-consumer-telehealth-service.

[2] "Digitalising healthcare for medical staff and patients," Telenor Group, July 5, 2018, https://www.telenor.com/media/press-release/digitalising-healthcare-for-medical-staff-and-patients/.

[3] See http://www.mytonic.com/en.

[4] Kathy Norcross Watts, "Helping Hands: WFBMC's Supporters of Health," June 28, 2017, https://www.journalnow.com/winstonsalemmonthly/features/helping-hands-wfbmc-s-supporters-of-health/article_1d3472ba-5c69-11e7-a1e8-7b1cc2a15a57.html.

[5] Ibid.

[6] Robert Wachter, *The Digital Doctor: Hope, Hype and Harm at the Dawn of Medicine's Computer Age* (New York: McGraw-Hill, 2015).

[7] Francis S. Collins, "Exceptional Opportunities in Medical Science: A View from The National Institutes of Health," *JAMA* 313, no.2 (2015):131-132, DOI: 10.1001/jama.2014.16736.

[8] Sarah Buhr, "Illumina wants to sequence your whole genome for $100," Tech Crunch, January 10, 2017, https://techcrunch.com/2017/01/10/illumina-wants-to-sequence-your-whole-genome-for-100/.

[9] See https://www.joinallofus.org/en/about.

[10] Teryl K. Nuckols et al., "The Shifting Landscape in Utilization of Inpatient, Observation, and Emergency Department Services Across Payers," *Journal of Hospital Medicine* 12, no.6 (2017): 443-446, DOI: 10.12788/jhm.p 51.

[11] J. Scott Ashwood, "Retail clinic visits for low-acuity conditions increase utilization and spending," *Health Affairs* 35, no.3 (2016):449-455.

[12] Rebecca Pifer, "Humana study touts telehealth cost cuts, with comparable follow-ups," Healthcare Dive, July 18, 2018, https://www.healthcaredive.com/news/humana-study-touts-telehealth-cost-cuts-with-comparable-follow-ups/527854/.

[13] See https://www.cms.gov/Newsroom/MediaReleaseDatabase/Press-releases/2018-Press-releases-items/2018-02-14.html.

[14] "2015 Comparative Price Report, Variation in Medical and Hospital Prices by Country," International Federation of Health Plans, accessed on January 30, 2018, https://fortunedotcom.files.wordpress.com/2018/04/66c7d-2015comparativepricereport09-09-16.pdf.

[15] Barry P. Bosworth, "Sources of Real Wage Stagnation," Brookings, December 22, 2014, https://www.brookings.edu/opinions/sources-of-real-wage-stagnation/.

[16] National Research Council and Committee on Population. *US health in international perspective: Shorter lives, poorer health.* (National Academies Press, 2013).

[17] Vasilis Kontis et al., "Future life expectancy in 35 industrialised countries: projections with a Bayesian model ensemble," The Lancet *389, no.10076 (2017): 1323-1335.*

[18] Anne Case and Sir Angus Deaton, "Mortality and morbidity in the 21st century," Brookings, March 23, 2017, https://www.brookings.edu/bpea-articles/mortality-and-morbidity-in-the-21st-century/.

[19] Gopal K. Singh et al., "Social Determinants of Health in the United States: Addressing Major Health Inequality Trends for the Nation. 1935-2016," *International Journal of MCH and AIDS* 6, no.2 (2017):139-164, DOI: 10.21106/ijma.236.

[20] Kadambini Tripathy, Tushar Nanda, and O.V. Sudharani, "The Influence of Environmental and Genetic Factors on Various Disorders and Diseases," *Journal of Genetic Syndromes & Gene Therapy* 2, no.1 (2011), DOI: 10.4172/2157-7412.S11-001.

[21] "Digitalising healthcare for medical staff and patients," Telenor Group, July 5, 2018, https://www.telenor.com/media/press-release/digitalising-healthcare-for-medical-staff-and-patients/.

[22] Manan Udayan Shah et al., "iPhone otoscopes: Currently available, but reliable for teleotoscopy in the hands of parents?," *International Journal of Pediatric Otorhinolaryngology* 106, (2018): 59-36.

[23] See Abrams K, Korba C, "Consumers are on board with virtual health options," at https://www2.deloitte.com/insights/us/en/industry/health-care/virtual-health-care-consumer-experience-survey.html?id=us:2em:3na:4di4631:5awa:6di:090618&ctr=textlink&sfid=003140000299CwJAAU

[24] See https://www.aapca1.org/sites/aapca1/files/downloads/sutter_health_formatted-telepsychiatry-_10.19.pdf.

[25] J. Michael McGinnis, Pamela Williams-Russo, and James R. Knickman, " The Case for More Active Policy Attention to Health Promotion," *Health Affairs* 21, no.2 (2002): 78-93, https://doi.org/10.1377/hlthaff.21.2.78.

[26] Robert L. Phillips, "International learning on increasing the value and effectiveness of primary care (I LIVE PC)." *The Journal of the American Board of Family Medicine* 25, no. Suppl 1: S2-S5, DOI: 10.3122/jabfm.2012.02.110198.

[27] Verbal communication, Kristi Henderson, Vice President of Patient Access and Care Delivery Transformation at Ascension, August 2018.

[28] See https://www.wired.com/2017/03/voice-is-the-next-big-platform-unless-you-have-an-accent/.

HEALTH CARE WITHOUT WALLS: INTRODUCTORY CHAPTER IN BRIEF

1. A health care system based on "Health Care Without Walls" could be construed as a system that came to people, meeting them where they are, in their homes, workplaces, or elsewhere in their communities—rather than expecting people to always go to it. It would be a health-inducing system that worked to keep people as healthy as possible, and, if people became ill because the system had failed to prevent it, would recognize that as a failure. It would also be as convenient and accessible as other elements of life that people now take for granted, such as sending money with an app on a mobile phone, or ordering groceries online.

2. NEHI, the Network for Excellence in Health Innovation, conducted a year-long investigation into the opportunities and challenges that confront Health Care Without Walls, aided by approximately 200 experts and health sector participants. In this report, it concludes that it is a national imperative to move more toward a system of Health Care Without Walls to capture a range of benefits—from vastly improved access to care for people living in underserved parts of the United States, to increased cost-efficiency in the provision of care.

3. Many different types of people could benefit from, and even thrive, in such an environment, ranging from relatively healthy consumers who need occasional access to the health care system, to individuals with serious health challenges, such as chronic illnesses like diabetes and heart disease, or mental and behavioral

health issues. NEHI has sketched a number of hypothetical scenarios in this report that suggest how various types of people and patients could benefit.

4. Multiple examples of more "distributed" or "virtual" care already exist, so a system of "Health Care Without Walls" is not a pipe dream. As the science fiction writer William Gibson once remarked, "The future is already here—it's just not very evenly distributed." A prominent example is the Kaiser Permanente health system, which now covers nearly 1 in every 30 Americans, in which 50 percent of the roughly 120 million patient encounters annually now take place over the phone, email, or video. The "digitization" of health care information over the past two decades has paved the way for increased use of distributed health care modalities.

5. Not all aspects of health care can or should be "delivered" outside of conventional institutional settings. Trauma centers, intensive care units, surgical settings and other places where "laying on of hands" occurs will not and should not disappear. "Distributed" health care outside of these settings will mainly be forms of health care that involve exchanges of information, which have moved to more virtual platforms in most other aspects of contemporary society already. As some observers have put it, the lag in adoption of technology into health care means that the system is one that delivers "Star Wars" medicine, but on a "Flintstones" delivery platform.

6. Nonetheless, NEHI found that substantial opportunities exist to equip health sector workers with technologies to advance more distributed care—so many that technology is clearly not the rate-limiting factor in the growth of Health Care Without Walls. Other trends under way in health care could also speed the evolution of more distributed care strategies, such as the growing use of "precision medicine," or health care that is to tailored to particular patients or groups of patients through such strategies as genetic or molecular profiling.

7. Certain negative trends under way in U.S. health and health care make moving to a system of more distributed health care especially urgent. The high costs and, in particular, the high prices within U.S. health care warrant the need to experiment with cost-saving strategies, such as reducing the high labor cost component of health care, or the costs of maintaining large physical footprints of health care institutions. Poor access in many communities to adequate care, and a maldistribution of care providers, demand strategies to make better use of the existing health care work force. And the poor and, in many instances, worsening health of much of the population also requires a focus on upstream drivers of poor health status—the social and economic determinants of health—and the movement of care outside the walls of health care in order to address them.

8. Despite the potential of Health Care Without Walls, multiple obstacles stand in the way. Current modes of paying for health care frequently do not support provision of more distributed care, and new payment models should be devised to support it. Regulatory constraints at the state and federal level pose challenges, and in many instances, regulatory structures will need to be revised to accommodate more distributed health care. Today's health care work force is not educated, trained, or equipped well to deliver more technology-driven care. Human factors—the myriad ways technology may or may not be designed to be used well by human beings, and how humans adopt and adjust to technology— may be either enablers or obstacles.

9. NEHI's report contains recommendations in all five of these areas—technology, work force, payment, regulation, and human factors. The recommendations are aimed at a diverse group of people and entities, including policy makers, technology developers and users, health care systems, payers, those in charge of educating and training tomorrow's health care workers, and other stakeholders. The recommendations are designed to expedite the appropriate movement to more distributed care and in essence, "predict" the future by creating it.

SCENARIO 1: A MAN SEEKING STATE-OF-THE-ART CANCER CARE IN A REMOTE SETTING

DAVE IS a 42-year-old man newly diagnosed with non-small cell lung cancer on Kodiak Island, Alaska, where he works as a natural scientist. His cancer was diagnosed via imaging and tumor biopsy at a critical access hospital on Kodiak. He now wants to get his genome and his tumor sequenced and determine the best course of treatment. He is a healthy, active man who has never smoked. He has moderate income, but would be financially strained if he had to travel many miles to a premier cancer center for a prolonged stay.

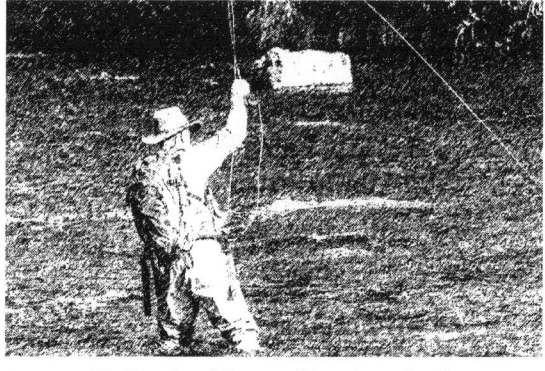

Although the most recent surveillance data shows lower age-adjusted cancer incidence in rural areas than metropolitan areas of the United States, death rates were higher in rural areas such as Kodiak Island (180 deaths per 100,000 persons) compared with urban areas (158 deaths per 100,000 persons [CDC, 2017]. Cancer death rates have fallen nationally but they have decreased at a slower pace in rural areas. What's more, there are several types of cancers with higher incidence rates in rural areas, including lung cancer, colorectal, and cervical cancers. Residence of rural areas frequently lack good access to cancer specialists and may have to travel hundreds, if not thousands, of miles for care.

Dave and his clinicians want to determine precise molecular pathway of his cancer, treat it optimally by seeking care from most knowledgeable clinicians possible, and treat him as close to home as possible. Dave values, above all, his quality of life and wants to preserve that as well.

At the same time, Dave can't imagine how, in the Internet age, he should not have access to the state-of-the art knowledge that exists in major cancer centers worldwide, and have that knowledge inform the care he receives on Kodiak Island.

Dave envisions the following scenario: His genome and his cancer's genome will be sequenced. That information, plus imaging and other test results, will be sent to oncologists at a premier cancer center on the mainland. Dave will have telehealth visits with the oncology team at the cancer center; the team will consult among themselves, and with the aid of the cognitive computing system, to determine the best care pathways, and then share that information with Dave. Assuming that he is a candidate for a targeted cancer therapy, that will be e-prescribed for him, dispatched from a specialty pharmacy in Seattle, Washington, and sent via express delivery to the critical access hospital on Kodiak Island. Various providers will hold virtual training sessions with the team at the critical access hospital on administration of the therapy, side effects to watch for, and other important matters. Dave will remain on Kodiak Island for now for his care, undergoing as much of it as possible on an outpatient basis.

All of the above in Dave's imagined care plan would be technically, and even technologically, possible. The forces that would stand in the way are inertia, friction in the system, and payment. Consider:

- Clinicians at the major cancer center would have to become licensed in Alaska in order to conduct telehealth consultations with Dave while he is on Kodiak Island.

- There would have to be agreements struck among health systems, as well as payers, not only about the amounts that would be paid for the various interventions, but how payments would be divided among the various care providers.

Dave and the head of the critical access hospital contact the chief of oncology at a premier mainland cancer center to discuss arrangements. They want to help, but immediately run into obstacles. At present, the center does not as a rule conduct telehealth visits to patients in other locations. There is no existing mechanism for sharing payment. The clinicians don't want to expend the effort to be licensed in Alaska, and they advise that taking the time to do so would only delay Dave's treatment.

Someday, they assure him, such telehealth-enabled provision of care will be routine. Someday, there may be national physician licensure that would obviate the need for physicians to obtain licenses in different states. Someday, enlightened payers may create payment models that would support such multi-site telehealth care. Just not now.

Dave, feeling defeated but resigned, books his travel to the mainland cancer center for additional exams and care. He prepares to draw down on his savings to meet transportation and lodging costs. He contacts relatives on the mainland to see if they can help to provide support while he undergoes treatment.

He thinks to himself: Surely, there is a better way.

◆ ◆ ◆

SCENARIO 2: AN ELDERLY WOMAN, LIVING ALONE, WITH MILD COGNITIVE IMPAIRMENT AND CHRONIC CONDITIONS

AS A YOUNG woman, Doris never imagined that she would live to her late 70s, and in quite this condition. Her husband, Joe, a former policeman, died several years ago; her daughter, Frances, now lives a few states away. Doris has grown somewhat frail, but she doesn't want to leave the Pittsburgh apartment where she has lived for the past quarter-century. She has a heart condition— atrial fibrillation; has been showing signs of mild cognitive impairment; and is somewhat lonely and mildly depressed. Doris is a so-called dual eligible, on both Medicare and Medicaid, and mostly lives on the income from Joe's Social Security.

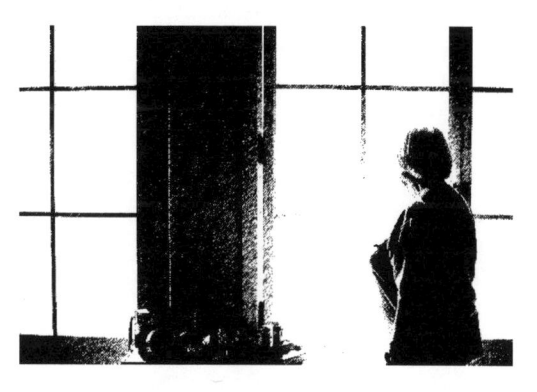

Between 10 percent and 20 percent of older U.S. adults are like Doris, in that they have mild cognitive impairment, or MCI, an intermediate state between normal cognition and dementia that can affect memory, speech, decision making, balance, and coordination. People with MCI have a high rate of progression to full-blown dementia over a relatively short period. An estimated 2.7 million to 6.1 million people in the United States have atrial fibrillation, the most common type of heart arrhythmia, and these numbers are expected to increase with the aging of the population. Because women live longer than men, more women than men experience AFib.

Frances wants Doris to move in with her, or to an assisted living facility, but Doris won't hear of it, and wants to live independently as long as possible. Frances has a long list of concerns: that, living alone, Doris could fall or sustain other injuries that could go unnoticed for days; that she may not eat regularly, or take her medication; that she might forget about and miss her medical appointments. Although Doris still has friends in her apartment building, Frances also worries that as these people age and die themselves, Doris may become increasingly isolated and lonely.

Doris's longtime cardiologist has advised that it's critical that Doris continue treatment for her heart condition. Frances and Doris's care team, which includes her primary care physician, all want to avoid having Doris make unnecessary visits to the hospital emergency department, or worse, be admitted for a hospital stay. Frances knows that her last hospitalization took a toll on Doris, as she lapsed at one point into delirium.

Frances has medical power of attorney, and in past hospitalizations, Doris and her daughter both agreed to a Do Not Resuscitate order for Doris that would bar "heroic" measures such as cardiopulmonary resuscitation, advanced cardiac life support, intubation, and tube feeding in the event that Doris underwent cardiac arrest or similar setback. Frances suspects that Doris would make the same choice if she were hospitalized again, but worries that if Doris is hospitalized and Frances isn't there, a DNR order may not be put in place, and Doris could receive aggressive and unwanted treatment.

Fortunately, Frances hears about an innovative PACE organization (Program of All-Inclusive Care of the Elderly) in Chicago that provides comprehensive medical and social services to frail, community-dwelling elderly individuals like Doris. This particular program has made a special commitment to adopting all manner of technological innovations in support of the care it provides. It also provides a home-based care coordination, with the support of an interdisciplinary team charged with meeting Doris's medical, psychosocial, and other needs.

Once Doris is enrolled in the program, a team of professionals meets with Doris and Frances to develop a personalized care plan. A home safety specialist tours Doris's home and corrects any issues that seem problematic, such as loose floor rugs. It is arranged that Doris will receive her primary care from a board-certified geriatrician, who will maintain close contact with Doris's existing cardiologist; she's also connected with a neurologist affiliated with the PACE program, who will monitor and possibly treat her mild cognitive impairment. When Doris needs to be seen in person, the program will dispatch a car and driver to pick Doris up to take her to her medical appointments, and is drawing up plans to use autonomous vehicles. A social worker will check in regularly via phone and a video screen to make sure Doris's other needs are being met. The social worker also lines up meals-on-wheels to deliver meals daily, as well as a home shopping service to deliver food and other supplies when Doris needs them.

Meanwhile, a technology coordinator who works for the PACE program installs a suite of tech-based services, and teaches Doris and Frances how to make the best use of them. An easily controlled video monitor allows for telehealth visits between Doris and her care providers, as well as Frances, and regular check-ins with the social worker. Doris gets an easy-to-use mobile phone especially made for seniors and learns how to have a FaceTime visit with Frances as well. Remote sensors are installed to keep track of Doris's movements and sleep patterns; they transmit data to the PACE program, where it is monitored to learn if anything is amiss. An automated pill box and dispenser sends alerts to both Frances and the PACE program if Doris doesn't take her medication. Doris can also use a voice activated task manager to call for rides or summon other assistance from the PACE program. The technology coordinator or an associate is on call 24/7 in case any difficulties arise with any of these technologies.

Despite all the technology, thanks the PACE program and her daughter's ongoing concern, Doris isn't lacking for human contact. A community health worker stops in to see Doris daily, and sometimes she and Doris both get on the video monitor to have a chat with Frances. They take a walk around the neighborhood or do some light exercises together. Frances knows how much her mother once enjoyed reading, and now makes sure she knows how to listen to audiobooks on her phone. At night Frances contacts her mother on the video monitor and they talk about the book that Doris is listening to, or catch up on the day's events.

Frances has no idea how long her mother will be able to stay mostly on her own this way. She's grateful that the PACE program is keeping a close eye on Doris to determine whether any change in Doris's cognitive status or overall health will necessitate a change. For now, at least, there is a solution that affords Doris the independence she still wants—and the peace of mind that Frances needs.

◆ ◆ ◆

CHAPTER 1: TECHNOLOGY AND HEALTH CARE WITHOUT WALLS

TECHNOLOGICAL INNOVATIONS—those available today and those likely to be available in 2025—have the clear potential to transform the health care landscape for patients, clinicians, caregivers, payers, and others.

Imagine, for example, a scenario in which an elderly patient with a heart condition gets an unexpected call while he is out shopping. His wrist monitor has transmitted a worrisome spike in his vital signs to his health system's communication center, and a digital virtual assistant immediately calls and suggests sending an autonomous (driverless) "medi-car" outfitted with medical sensors and other testing and communication devices to further assess his condition. After the virtual assistant receives and analyzes the results of additional tests performed in the car, it triggers a video consultation with an on-call physician, who has access to the patient's medical records and the data from the medi-car tests, and who determines what further actions are needed.

The technology underlying this scenario—the remote sensors, the autonomous car, and immediate access to the patient's records and the data just generated by medi-car's medical devices—is technology that exists today. It doesn't need to be invented—just adopted and put into use as described. Already, systems such as the Veterans Administration and Kaiser Permanente (which crafted the hypothetical scenario above),[29] among others, are delivering health care through technology-enabled telemedicine; replacing many physical visits with various types of "e-visits"; shifting care from traditional settings such as hospitals and physicians' offices to patients' homes and work sites; and exploring deployment of an array of other technologies, including remote monitoring of patients' vital signs, various "smart" devices, and computerized physician decision support enhanced by technologies such as artificial intelligence, data sciences, machine learning, natural language processing, and data analytics.

Such technologies hold the promise of more effective ways to predict, diagnose, and treat disease, enabled by collection of personalized data (from wearable sensors, smart phones, genomics, and other data sources) and the use of artificial intelligence, machine learning, and data analytics. The beginnings of this technological transformation of health care are already evident in the home and in other settings.

Internet of Things (IoT)

For example, the explosive growth of access to the Internet and to the "Internet of Things" (IoT)—the myriad devices wirelessly connected through the Internet, including many with health-related applications—represents "a formidable technologic force that makes medicine's democratization more likely and more powerful," notes Eric Topol, MD, director of the Scripps Translational Science Institute in La Jolla, Calif., in his 2015 book, *The Patient Will See You Now*.[30] Topol cites projections of 28 billion to 50 billion connected devices by 2020, with the average person having 6 to 7 such devices. Although more recent estimates are generally closer to 30 million than 50 million connected devices, it's clear that connected medical devices such as wearable and implanted biosensors will play an increasing role in health care.

Today, remote sensors provide data about sleep and activity patterns, blood pressure, weight, and oxygen and glucose levels of elderly individuals living at home for round-the-clock monitoring by nurses and data specialists. An ingestible sensor in the first digital pill, recently approved by the Food and Drug Administration, can notify physicians if and when a patient takes the medication. This device may help address the issue of nonadherence—patients not taking their medication as prescribed—which experts estimate results in nearly 125,000 deaths and 10% of hospitalizations annually, at a cost of $100 billion–$289 billion.[31] Researchers at Stanford are conducting the Apple Heart study, an effort to determine if an app for the Apple watch can detect abnormal heart rhythms, such as those associated with an increased risk for blood clots and strokes. In fact, the Apple watch newly released to the public in September 2018 contains FDA-approved technology enabling users to take an echocardiogram of their hearts.

Artificial Intelligence, Machine Learning, and Related Technologies

Artificial intelligence (AI), data science, and related technologies enable computers and computerized devices to perform tasks that normally require human intelligence, and to "learn" and adapt their functions when exposed to more data. These technologies are expected to radically reshape multiple industries, including various aspects of health care. AI has been described as a "collective term for computer systems that can sense their environment, think, learn, and take action in response to what they're sending and their objectives." [32] Potential applications in health care range from "smarter" scheduling of health care appointments, to enhancing diagnostic capacity, to "virtual" drug discovery and development [33]. (For a fuller discussion of AI in health care, see the report "Artificial Intelligence for Health and Health Care" by the JASON Group of scientific advisers to the federal government.) [34]

For example, many of the tasks that radiologists and pathologists now perform, such as screening for lung cancer on CT scans or determining a lung tumor's grade and stage, can be done as well (and sometimes better) by computers.[35] Ultimately, the goal of applying this technology to pathology and radiology is to free up these specialists for more cognitively complex tasks that cannot be done as well by an AI/machine system, including interpreting data and advising on next steps for managing a patient's condition.

As these technologies are developed further, they will increasingly support care that is provided in remote settings, such as homes. For example, CloudUPDRS, a smartphone app, monitors such symptoms of Parkinsons disease as tremor and uneven gait patterns, and employs an AI/machine learning algorithm to differentiate actual symptoms from erroneous signals such as a dropped phone. The tool enables Parkinson's patients to perform in-home testing and feed the information to their care providers, as will become more commonplace with other disease conditions over time. (See JASON report, supra.)

Smart robots are expected to be widely deployed in health care. For example, they may be used to help alleviate the social isolation experienced by many older adults—a problem that research suggests may contribute to health ills of elderly individuals, including higher levels of inflammation and stress hormones, impaired immunity, and increased risk of heart disease, stroke, and premature death. A device called ElliQ, which won a "Best of Innovation" award at CES 2018, the annual consumer technology show in Las Vegas, is designed to encourage older adults to keep active and engaged. The AI/machine learning-driven device, equipped with cameras, a removable tablet, and a smart speaker that can move to convey body language and light up to indicate that it is "paying attention" to a user, actually "learns" the user's habits and preferences. In addition to providing reminders about appointments or taking medications, it can also send messages to ride-hailing apps, proactively ask questions, or suggest music, videos, or physical activities, such as going for a walk.

Technological Benefits

All of these technologies, including digital tools and new channels for delivering health care services in a system built on "Health Care Without Walls" concepts, offer potentially large benefits to individuals and to the nation. Put simply, the vision within reach is of a health care system that is far more accessible and convenient, improves quality of care, removes some of the friction in health care, makes better use of clinicians, potentially lowers the cost of care, and offers a host of other benefits as well.

More distributed and accessible care

Technologies such as smartphones, apps, and remote sensors are already shifting care-related tasks and services outside of hospitals, doctor's offices, and other health care facilities. The shift makes it possible to meet patients where they are, including at home, in the work place, and in other community settings. This transition would particularly benefit underserved and/or vulnerable populations, including rural populations, who may struggle with access issues, including transportation; people such as the frail elderly; and some people with physical or intellectual disabilities who may also lack mobility or means of transport.

Greater convenience for consumers

Increased access to care on demand and medical services that can be delivered to homes or nonclinical locations translates to time and transportation savings for patients. The University of Virginia Medical Center in Charlottesville, for example, which offers telemedicine in 60 specialties and subspecialties, estimates that it has spared patients more than 17 million miles of driving to the medical center to obtain care.

Better quality of care

Factors such as improved access to care; more precise digital profiles of a patient's disease susceptibilities and health status; access to preventive care that averts costly care down the road; and devices that allow routine monitoring of a patient's condition, such as hypertension, and follow-up and interventions when needed, all make it possible to anticipate problems in patients' care and to act swiftly to address them. With telehealth, people with rare conditions can more easily consult specialists with particular expertise in their conditions. Technology-enabled care can also curb unnecessary care and reduce medical errors. Artificial-intelligence-enabled digital pathology—when, through a technology known as virtual microscopy, tissue samples on slides are digitized so that they can be analyzed using computer algorithms—in theory will enable diagnosis of cancers at earlier stages and more precise targeting of treatments.[36]

Managing chronic illness and avoiding unnecessary care

Devices and analytic tools may help predict an impending episode of illness (such as a depressive episode or an asthma attack) and allow for early intervention and avoidance of hospitalization. For example, Internet-enabled scales can weigh patients and transfer information about their weight remotely. Such systems are already being used to monitor patients with congestive heart failure (CHF), providing an early indication that they are retaining fluid, that their condition has been exacerbated for some reason, and that some change in treatment or diet is warranted.

Lower costs

Similarly, digital technologies can reduce costs by curbing unnecessary care and improving management of chronic diseases such as diabetes and asthma. In addition to remote monitoring, such as that described above with CHF patients, such technologies can help avert emergency department visits and hospitalization; reduce the time clinicians spend on nonclinical tasks such as updating medical records; and improve the diagnostic process through use of clinical support tools based on data input and analysis. All of these results lead to care that is less costly or more cost-effective and efficient than it might be otherwise.

Less "friction" in the health care system

Care that is delivered virtually, such as through telehealth, can avoid physical visits to care providers and the accompanying time, expense, absenteeism, lost productivity, and delayed access to care that can be associated with them. For example, telehealth nurse practitioners are stationed in the emergency departments of 17 rural Mississippi hospitals to treat patients via a multidisciplinary team that includes a certified emergency medicine physician on the University of Mississippi Medical Center (UMMC) campus in Jackson. Through a service called UMMC 2, Mississippi state employees and their dependents can receive telehealth services from UMMC clinicians from their own homes and work sites.[37]

Better use of the existing corps of providers

Digital tools can support physicians and other clinicians in "working at the top of their licenses," as well as assist clinicians and nonclinical staff in doing other tasks at the top of their abilities while avoiding more menial work. For example, documenting patient encounters—the process of adding information gleaned from visits with patients to electronic health records—is tedious and time-consuming, and could be streamlined with speech recognition and natural language processing technology—which could also be analyzed for thick data patterns. Patients could experience longer encounters—including virtual ones—with less-harried providers, and clinicians could spend more time with patients when warranted, especially those with more complex conditions.

Reduced clinician "burnout"

In addition to helping transfer nonclinical tasks such as documentation to non-clinicians, the use of artificial intelligence, data science, and other digital tools, coupled with new work force arrangements that include new types of data specialists, could help to reduce "data fatigue" by filtering the tsunami of data necessary to support clinical decision-making. For example, using digital tools to sift through data in real time to recognize patterns can help identify patients whose condition is deteriorating and alert staff that closer management and intervention are needed. Sepsis-related mortality rates dropped by about 53 percent at an Alabama hospital after a computerized surveillance algorithm was put into place and hospital staff were trained about sepsis and the use of the alerting system. Real-time analytics alerted clinicians to new diagnoses of sepsis or worsening vital signs, and the system also issued advice alerts with information about evidence-based care for sepsis.[38] Through

AI technologies, patients' records can be monitored, and proposed treatments identified, even as clinicians take their first steps into an exam room to see patients.[39]

Better care coordination

Central to care coordination is communication among various members of a patient's care team. Technologies such as electronic heath record (EHR) systems can automatically distribute information to the team while still maintaining patient privacy. Health information exchange and EHR interoperability enable providers in different health care systems to share information about patients' histories, including past and present treatment, laboratory test results, medications, and allergies. There is a growing movement to grant patients direct access to EHRs, perhaps by creating a set of personal health records that they would control. Such PHRs would in theory store data from all prior health care visits as well as patient-generated health data from personal health trackers, for example; patients could then share it with their providers and family care givers as they chose.

Telehealth technology also can transmit data from biometric devices, along with responses (by patients or caregivers) to questions. On the receiving end, software can identify changes in a patient's condition and flag it for review by a clinician or care coordinator, who then determines if additional assessment or actions are needed to address the patient's condition.

Enabling precision medicine

Collecting, synthesizing, and assessing massive amounts of data relating to the genome and other "omes," such as the proteome or microbiome, holds the potential to help clinicians make more precise diagnoses and prognoses. These masses of data are also expected to inform predictive analytics that can help identify people who are at risk for certain diseases or who are likely to need specific types of care. For such patients, preventive measures and other early interventions may be identified, and closer surveillance could help detect disease at an early stage.

Universalized and "democratized" knowledge and expertise

In an era where nearly any patient, anywhere, could go online to access information about state-of-the art medical care for a given condition, many of these same patients lack direct access to the specialists who have generated that medical knowledge, as well as to other top-quality care providers. The internet should render this inequity obsolete. There is no technological reason that a patient almost anywhere in the world could not have access to a top-ranked specialist in any medical field and to his or her knowledge. Technology holds the potential to "democratize" health care and enable the spread of knowledge almost everywhere.

Improved public health

Social media and other technologies can help track infectious disease outbreaks or predict possible complications based on environmental news (such as risks posed by poor air quality for people with compromised lung function). For example, although the Google Flu Trends (GFT) experiment—an attempt to track influenza prevalence by tracking search for flu-related information on Google—was widely deemed a failure due to poor methodology, "Google's sequel to GFT, done right, could serve as a model for collaboration around big data for the public good," wrote David Lazer and Ryan Kennedy, two researchers who led a team that critiqued the GFT in a 2014 article in the journal Science.[40,41]

Advancing population health strategies

Technology can help address social and economic determinants such as transportation issues, food and housing insecurity, and other upstream drivers of health and poor health. For example, integrating health and health-care related information from a range of sources—electronic health records, claims data from payers, patient data from providers (including data from patient questionnaires asking about social determinants), demographic data, environmental data, and data from activity trackers and remote monitoring devices—could help identify factors affecting the health of individuals and populations and point to useful interventions. Such information can be used to link patients with government programs and other resources such as housing, food banks, and utility reconnection services. Telehealth technology can help overcome barriers to accessing care, such as transportation issues. Social media can be used to help identify and track infectious disease outbreaks, such as influenza, measles, or foodborne illness.

Organizations Venturing Into Health Care Without Walls

As noted, a number of health systems have already ventured into more distributed care to take advantage of the many benefits described above.

- In 2015, Kaiser Permanente's more than 10 million enrollees (at that time) experienced more than half of their interactions with clinicians virtually (via such means as e-visits, emails, and phone calls). The organization projects that e-visits alone will exceed in-person visits by 2020. In 2018, Kaiser Permanente says it is on track to have 60 percent of total patient encounters within its system occur virtually—either by phone, email, or telehealth visit. Kaiser is studying the implications of this shift, but early evidence suggests great patient satisfaction, among other positive outcomes.

- The Veterans' Health Administration, the largest integrated health system in the United States, has operated telehealth and multiple other digital services for its patients for more than a decade. Now organized under the umbrella of Connected Care, these services include both home- and clinic-based consumer-facing telehealth, as well as store-and-forward technologies, which involve the acquisition and storing of clinical information (for example, radiological images that are then forwarded to or retrieved by another site for clinical evaluation.) These technologies can be used in connection with others offered to veterans by the VA, such as My HealtheVet, the VA's Personal Health Record. HealtheVet allows veterans to record diet, exercise, and health history; send a message to their VA care team; refill VA medications; track VA appointments; and review notes from their last clinic visit. Another VA capability, VA Mobile Health, develops health apps for Veterans and VA care teams that increase access, communication and coordination of care for Veterans.[42]

- The Mount Sinai Health System in New York City offers selected patients with certain acute conditions the opportunity to avoid or be sent home from the emergency department for "hospitalization at home." The system tested the approach in a three-year demonstration project through the Centers for Medicare and Medicaid Services' Innovation Center that ended in September 2017; Mount Sinai patients who were "hospitalized" at home received daily (or more frequent) visits from a clinician, who checked vital signs and administered some medications, such as infusions. Laboratory services, intravenous medications, and necessary equipment also were brought to patients' homes. Following the hospitalization period, patients were also closely monitored during a 30-day post-acute care transition component. Compared to a control group of hospital inpatients, patients who were "hospitalized" at home had shorter lengths-of-stay; lower hospital readmission rates within 30 days after discharge; fewer re-visits to emergency departments and admissions to skilled nursing facilities; and higher patient satisfaction.[43] Costs were also lower, by about 20%.

Mount Sinai is now expanding its program by partnering with commercial payers, Medicare Advantage plans, and other entities, including Contessa Health (a health care company that manages acute-care services at home through prospective bundled payment arrangements). Elsewhere, physician group Atrius in Massachusetts has also launched a hospital-at-home programs in tandem with a private developer of such programs, the Medically Home Group, as has the Marshfield Clinic in Wisconsin.

- CVS Health, Target, and Walgreens have opened retail clinics in thousands of stores nationwide. And under its planned acquisition of health insurer Aetna, CVS plans to transform many of its stores into "health hubs," offering some on-site care, but also connecting to consumers' homes and to other health care providers via telemedicine and other technologies.

- Reintroducing the house call to health care, companies such as Heal, Pager, Curbside Care, and others have emerged to meet consumer desire for on-demand health care services provided by physicians or nurses in the patient's home.

- In a pilot program called UberHEALTH, HealthMap Vaccine Finder (an organization that offers a searchable online map to find local vaccine providers) teamed up with the ride-hailing company Uber for a one-day opportunity in four U.S. cities. Users could request an Uber car with a nurse to come to their home or office to administer up to 10 flu shots for free. More than 40 percent of requesters had never received a flu shot before the event, and more than 90 percent of responders to a survey after the event said that the delivery aspect of the program was important. UberHEALTH had a similar event in collaboration with the Apollo hospital chain in Hyderabad, India. This one-day effort (held on World Health Day), involved sending an Uber car with an Apollo practitioner to homes or offices to collect blood samples for testing for diabetes and thyroid disease.

    The ride-hailing companies Uber and Lyft are also working with hospitals and health insurers to increase access to nonemergency health care for patients with transportation issues.

- Use of remote monitoring of seniors in independent living is already growing and is likely to expand. LivingWell@Home, a service of Evangelical Lutheran Good Samaritan Society, uses remote sensors to track sleep and activity patterns and telehealth technology to monitor blood pressure, weight, and oxygen and glucose levels; the data are monitored 24/7 by registered nurses and data specialists.

Other services are being offered entirely online, such as online psychotherapy on demand through audio, video, or text. For example, Big White Wall is a digital and behavioral health and well-being service facilitated by health care professionals, which was designated a High Impact Innovation by England's National Health Service (NHS) and formally endorsed by the NHS in 2015. In 2014, it expanded to the United States, but has since ceased operations in this country even though it remains available to users in England, including through the NHS.[44]

Barriers and Challenges

However great the promise, developing and incorporating telehealth and other digital technologies and related innovations into health care face an array of challenges. Among these are cost, payment, and reimbursement issues; federal and state regulations tailored to older modes of health care, and issues of privacy and data security; a variety of issues affecting the current work force; human factors that can impede the uptake and use of technology, and a lack of understanding on the part of technology developers and entrepreneurs of the challenges faced by clinicians, consumers, and payers. These challenges are discussed at length in subsequent chapters of this report.

Other challenges speak to the difficulties of incorporating new technologies and approaches into what is already a complex enterprise. For example, sponsors of hospital-at-home programs cite the effort of creating a "just-in-time" supply chain, in which the types of medical products and other supplies that are normally delivered in bulk to a hospital are instead delivered in vastly smaller quantities, and on a real-time basis, directly to patients' homes.

What's more, the history of adoption of information technology into health care is riddled with examples of hugely expensive projects gone awry—and health systems still have legacy information systems installed that make transition to more modern systems difficult. In the United States, as well as in other countries such as Britain, the adoption of electronic health records technology has been plagued by huge costs, a perceived lack of usability, and to date in the United States, failure to achieve system-wide interoperability. A major lesson is that any new information and technology systems that are adopted must be flexible and adaptable, and that organizations should be careful to make well thought out strategic investments in this all-important arena.

`All this said, building a technology-enabled health care system with its many benefits by 2025 is feasible. However, it will require a sense of urgency and determination to work through the many barriers standing in the way. Many of the innovations characterizing "Health Care Without Walls," such as telehealth, would already be in broader use today if various barriers to their development and dissemination had previously been addressed. Failing to seize the opportunity to overcome the obstacles to achieving this vision would be an enormous missed opportunity, for patients and for the nation.

Participants in the Health Care Without Walls initiative believe that it is essential to advance not only the individual technologies, but also the overall vision of a health care system that better connects individuals, populations, and their care providers in direct pursuit of better health and care. "The care you need, when and where you need it" is the ultimate goal; the technology is just one of the vitally important means toward that end.

Goals of the Technology Work Stream

The Technology Work Stream of the Health Care Without Walls initiative was charged with examining current and future technologies that could realistically be in place, and widely used, in the U.S. health care system in 2025, assuming that barriers to their development and dissemination were addressed. Among the work stream's goals were the following:

- Create a vision of the future through a set of scenarios depicting care options for various patients and populations, and detailing how care could be delivered to them with the aid of an array of technologies.

- Identify barriers to deployment and take-up of technologies, in conjunction with the other work streams.

- Draft recommendations for changes in public policy and within health care organizations, payers, and others, to support the 2025 technology vision and stimulate advocacy to achieve this vision.

Health Care Technologies

Common elements

Although there is a range of technologies that would advance the Health Care Without Walls vision, work stream participants argued that the most useful technologies will have common elements or general unifying themes, as follows:

- **Usability.** Technologies should be easy to use and "frictionless" for users, seamlessly integrated into their lives so that they become an almost invisible part of the health care journey. An analogy would be the relationship that users have with a smartphone, an extremely complex device with sophisticated technology that the typical user does not need to understand in order to use effectively. Technologies should be viewed as the engine under the hood of the car—essential, but largely out of sight for typical users.

- **Transparency.** Although usability is important for typical use of digital technology, such technologies also should be transparent, allowing those with more expertise, including end users, to "interrogate" the system to examine the underlying digital coding and algorithms. Such examination would facilitate investigation of any biases and limitations of a technology and development of ways to improve it or tailor it to the needs of different users.

- **Interoperability.** A necessary element of a frictionless and seamless health care experience is the ability of systems and devices to exchange data under open, common, and widely shared data standards; to allow data to follow the patient; and to present data in such a way that they are clearly understood and actionable for users. Interoperability is an important element for not just patients, but for all users, including clinicians and caregivers.

- **A commitment to data sharing and information exchange.** Technology Work Stream members stressed that realizing the potential of digital technologies to promote distributed care and optimize health system performance will require a more collaborative open-source approach to sharing patient data (while preserving patient confidentiality). Interoperability is one necessary component for the seamless flow of data. Equally important, providers, payers, technology companies, app developers, and others should commit to a more collaborative approach to sharing patient data while preserving patient confidentiality, and also should exchange such data to support the coordination of care.

- **Privacy and security.** At the same time as systems must promote appropriate data sharing, they must also guard against exposing patients' personally identifiable health information and must maintain the security of these data. This difficult balancing act—promulgating appropriate data sharing while also guarding privacy and security—is discussed at length in subsequent chapters of this volume.

- **Integration and convergence of all components.** Technologies should enable care in a way that all components are seamlessly connected. For example, a patient at home should be able to use an online app to summon a provider to the home; the visiting provider should be able to use a point-of-care diagnostic or an ultrasound device; and the data from these activities should be able to be uploaded directly into an electronic health record or other repository of patient data.

- **Ubiquitous Internet access.** Universal access to affordable, fast, broadband Internet by 2025 is essential to the Health Care Without Walls 2025 vision. (See regulatory chapter for discussion on the barriers, and recommendations for achieving this objective).

- **Other conceptual features.** Technology Work Stream participants felt that other key features are necessary to ensure that a technology-based system is truly patient-centric. Technologies should be designed and implement in ways that "do no harm," in which safety and ethical principles are embedded in the system.

Glossary: Technologies and Areas of Application

Below is a broad, albeit not exhaustive, list of technologies and critical elements of technologies that are in use today and that could be more widely used throughout U.S. health care in 2025.

- **Apps (short for Applications).**

Mobile or Web-based health and fitness applications used on smartphones, tablets, and computers. An integrated suite of apps can work together to help patients manage a health condition. Such apps are even more effective when they have access to all of a consumer's health data made possible by a personal health record. An example is Rango, an online program to help people with HIV manage their own health; it promotes treatment adherence and provides support groups. Other apps can

- o Allow patients to upload information (such as blood pressure or blood glucose readings) for providers to review.

- o Help patients record and track a variety of personal health-related data (physical activity; calories and nutrient intake; sleep; blood pressure, blood glucose, heart rate, and other metrics) and issue prompts, such as reminders for taking medications.

- o Assemble data uploaded to providers that can be tracked and assessed for trends (such as weight, blood pressure, blood glucose, mood, exercise), which can signify that medical intervention may be needed.

- o Provide data for analytics, including predictive analytics.

- **Artificial Intelligence (AI) Data Sciences, and Machine Learning.**

  The goal of this area of technology is to simulate human thought processes in a computerized model. Currently, people often use the term artificial intelligence (AI), which encompasses a number of areas (including machine learning, natural language processing, and other fields), broadly and imprecisely. When applied to medicine and health care, these technologies often involve the use of algorithms with machine learning capabilities (self-learning systems, algorithms that can recognize patterns and learn from and make predictions based on data). AI/machine learning can be used to help assess and predict health care needs and problems and to suggest solutions.

  Current and potential applications are legion, and include monitoring emotional responses, predicting episodes of depression and anxiety, and alerting providers; recognizing and understanding human speech; interpreting complex data; computer-aided detection; computer-aided diagnosis; decision support tools; and much more. In general, these technologies are considered relatively new in health care, and there is debate as to how soon they will be in broad use in various areas and in how effective they will be. But there is little doubt that they will play a growing role in health care.

- **Advanced Portable Screening Technologies.**

These tools, such as handheld ultrasound devices or smartphones equipped with echocardiogram technology, have very nearly made stethoscopes obsolete. The equivalent of devices that just a few years ago were mainly available in hospitals or other advanced health care settings are now available on these and other handheld devices.

- **Augmented Reality (see also Virtual Reality).**

Computer-generated images that are superimposed on an individual's view of the real world, thus providing a composite view. An example might be training a patient in how to help manage disease by superimposing on a picture of the patient's body an image of an internal organ or organ system, and displaying the impact of correctly taking medication.

- **Autonomous (Self-driving) Cars.**

These vehicles could transport patients for in-person medical services or bring medical personnel, services, equipment, or supplies to homes or other nonclinical sites. Car technology could include biosensors to measure parameters such as temperature, heart rate, and respiration.

- **Blockchain Technology.**

This technology (currently used for financial transactions, such as for Bitcoin) is seen as a way to use encryption and decentralized databases to securely share medical records, protect them from hackers, allow providers to use the data without incompatibility problems, and provide patients with more control over their health information.

- **Clinical Decision Support.**

Use of AI/machine learning and other tools to help diagnose and treat illness, increase efficiency, and reduce errors.

- **Care Management Systems, Population Management Systems.**

  These systems use digital technology to manage health of defined populations, one of the key components of the "triple aim" approach for optimizing performance of a health system (improving the experience of care, improving the health of populations, and reducing per capita costs of health care). Collection, integration, and analysis of large data sets, such as clinical and claims data, can help identify populations with modifiable risks; other tools can help identify and direct and coordinate the appropriate interventions to patients with specific health risks and conditions.

- **Cloud.**

  A vast network of remote servers around the globe that are connected and meant to operate as a single ecosystem. These servers are designed to either store and manage data, run applications, or deliver content or a service such as streaming videos, web mail, office productivity software, or social media. Instead of accessing files and data from a local or personal computer, an individual or entity accesses them online from any Internet-capable device, and the information is available anywhere and at any time.

- **Cloud computing.**

  The delivery of computing services—servers, storage, databases, networking, software, analytics, and more—over the Internet ("the cloud"). Cloud computing eliminates the capital expense of buying hardware and software and setting up and running on-site datacenters—the racks of servers, the round-the-clock electricity for power and cooling, the IT experts for managing the infrastructure.

- **Customer (Patient) Relationship Management Systems.**

  Use of practices and technologies by providers to engage patients and develop long-term relationships with them. Such technologies, including social media, online portals, data analytics, and other tools, have been successfully used by non-health care companies to collect and analyze information to optimize work flow and identify and anticipate customer needs. When applied to the health care arena, digital technologies could help patients manage their care between visits with clinicians, such verifying their understanding of and adherence to a recent change in their treatment plan (and triggering subsequent involvement by a care team member if the patient's response suggests intervention is needed). Patient health portals can enhance patients' relationship with providers by allowing them to request appointments and medication refills, access and fill out pre-visit forms, pay bills, and receive communications about lab results from their provider.[45]

- **Data Lake.**

A centralized repository where structured and unstructured data can be stored, at any scale. Organizations can use the data to run different types of analytics—from dashboards and visualizations to big data processing, real-time analytics, and machine learning to guide better decisions.

- **Data Warehouse.**

A large store of data accumulated from a wide range of sources within a company and used to guide management decisions.

- **Diagnostics, either Remote or Point of Care.**

  Examples include:
  - A "tricorder"-like device that includes sensors and an AI/machine learning engine to diagnose common conditions.
  - Point-of-care tests.
  - Self-administered tests, such as HemoLink, an FDA-approved needle-free blood draw test device.

- **Drones.**

These have the potential to speed delivery of medical supplies such as pharmaceuticals to remote or relatively inaccessible areas, or in highly populated areas at times when traffic conditions would impede quick delivery.

- **Electronic Health Records (EHRs).**

A digital technology that documents an individual's medical and treatment history (including diagnoses, laboratory data and radiology reports and images, allergies, medications, and other information), as well as provides a broader view of a patient's health and care. EHRs have the potential to improve patient care. Ideally, EHRs enable authorized providers to add information and manage the EHR in a digital format that can be shared with other providers across more than one health care organization, allow access to evidence-based tools that help clinicians make decisions about a patient's care, and automate and streamline workflow. At present, however, in the U.S. health care system, true interoperability of EHRs—the ability to exchange data and information seamlessly—has not yet been achieved.

- **Fifth Generation (5G) Cellular Service:**

The next generation of cellular networks that will deliver data at extremely fast speeds and open up a range of new applications, beginning in many U.S. cities in 2018. Telephones compatible with 5G technology are expected to become broadly available in the U.S. in 2019. Data transmitted over 5G cellular lines will travel nearly instantaneously, and will be able to be downloaded in huge amounts at very fast speeds. 5G technology will allow many more internet-enabled objects to connect to cellular towers, including remote monitoring devices, other medical devices and home appliances.

- **Health Information Technology.**

An umbrella term that includes such digital technologies as electronic health records, which document a person's health care experiences. It is broadly agreed that EHR's should be accessible to all members of a patient's care team, although at present, true interoperability of EHRs—the ability to share data and information seamlessly—is lacking in the U.S. health care system. Secure communications may also take place via "trust frameworks" and blockchain technology (see "Blockchain"). EHRs are also a potential source of data for patient registries, predictive analytics, and a wide variety of research efforts.

- **Interoperable technology.**

Interoperability refers to the ability of systems and devices to exchange data and information under open, common, and widely shared data standards; to allow data to follow the patient; and to present data in such a way that they are clearly understood and actionable for users. Although interoperability is considered a necessary element of a frictionless and seamless health care experience, true interoperability for a key element in health care, electronic health records, is lacking.

- **Machine Learning.**

    A subset of AI, machine learning refers to self-learning algorithms that enable digital devices to analyze and detect patterns in existing data, identify similar patterns and improve performance when exposed to new data, and make data-driven predictions.

- **Medical Internet of Things.**

    An estimated 30 billion connected devices globally are predicted by 2020, about 6-7 digital tools on average per person worldwide. Many will be collecting billions of personalized bits of data, including about individuals' "-omes" (such as the genome, epigenome, microbiome, proteome, etc.); these data can be analyzed and provide the opportunity to monitor and make predictions about a patient's health.

- **Patient Registries.**

    These online data platforms contain patient data, including data already stored in EHRs. They can be tapped for information to be used in conjunction with predictive analytics to help prioritize care for patients (such as which individuals need to be seen more often). Data mined from patient registries also can help payers, providers, patients, biopharmaceutical companies, and others understand the value of specific treatments.

- **Personal Health Record** (as distinct from Electronic Health Record):

    A record or health record bank that is consumer-centered and consumer-controlled and that would gather all of a patient's treatment history and relevant data. Patients and consumers could then make their complete, unified, lifetime health record available to other providers, family caregivers, and even medical research organizations of their choosing.

- **Personalized/Precision Medicine.**

    Health care that is tailored to the individual through use of technologies such as genetic screening, "omics," data collected via remote sensors, and predictive analytics.

- **Predictive Analytics.**

    Extracting information from existing data sets to determine patterns and predict future outcomes and trends. For example, software that analyzes clinical data in electronic health records and claims data could identify patients at high risk for costly interventions in the near term and trigger needed follow-up clinical visits and testing.

- **Remote Monitors (also see "Sensors").**

    Internet-enabled devices in the home or other non-clinical settings. Other devices can gather and process environmental data that affects health (such as air quality, pollen counts).

- **Robotics.**

    Physically assistive robots could visit an individual at home to deliver medications or perform tests; robots in the home could perform certain tasks. Socially assistive robots could engage patients with conditions such as Alzheimer disease and help prevent social isolation in mobility-challenged patients.

- **Sensors (also see "remote monitors").**

    These devices include wearables, implantables, and ingestibles, and can be used in remote monitoring tools that can transmit information directly into an electronic health record or an individual's personal health record. Some measure biological signs (such as temperature, blood pressure, heart rate, respiration); others measure other factors that affect health (such as smart pills that signal when a medication has been ingested). Certain implantable devices, such as insulin pumps and left-ventricular assist devices, will also increasingly communicate wirelessly with various sensing devices such as continuous glucose monitoring and pulmonary artery pressure monitoring systems. Automobile-based technologies are likely to include biosensors to measure temperature, heart rate, and respiration.

- **Telehealth and Telemedicine (terms used interchangeably).**

    Use of digital information and communications technologies, including mobile devices such as smartphones and tablets, as well as home or desktop computers, for patient care, interaction between patients and providers, among patients (for example, through online support groups), and among providers, all remotely. Telemedicine consultations between providers and patients could be especially valuable in rural and underserved settings and for vulnerable populations, like the frail elderly. Telehealth and telemedicine are often used in concert with other technologies, and encompass a broad range of applications:

    o Real-time video interactions, such as for virtual visits with providers and health coaching.

    o Access to an online patient portal for communicating with a patient's care team to schedule appointments, request refills, view test results, and access health records.

    o Remote monitoring, in conjunction with such technologies as wearable sensors or other devices that measure and transmit information such as heart rate, blood glucose, physical activity, and sleep patterns.

    o Virtual consultations between primary care physicians and specialists.

    o Delivery of health-related education and coaching, such as targeted text messages to encourage healthy behaviors.

    o Supporting medical education for providers.

    o Supporting public health activities, such as health alerts.

- **Teleradiology.**

    Increasingly used by hospitals, clinics, and others, often driven by lack of on-site radiology staff. In the future, however, the expectation is that most images will be "read" via technology that features AI/machine learning and deep learning, a subtype of AI/machine learning in which the software tries to simulate the brain's immense array of neurons in an artificial neural network.

- **3-D Printing.**

    Increasingly small and portable printers may make it possible to "print" assistive devices tailored for patients in the home, office, or other non-clinical setting.

- **Virtual Reality (see also Augmented Reality).**

    The computer-generated simulation of three-dimensional images or environments that individuals can interact with by using special electronic equipment, such as helmets or headsets with screens or gloves equipped with sensors. Applications are innumerable, but could include treatment of patients with post-traumatic stress disorder through so-called exposure therapy; conducting support groups for patients with adjustable level of anonymity; or even "gamification" of rehabilitation activities.

- **Voice Recognition and Interactive Voice Response (IVR).**

    These technologies support a broad variety of health care–related interactions, saving time and making interactions more efficient and frictionless. They hold the potential to sharply reduce the time it takes for tasks like documentation and automating and integrating the physician's diagnosis to an e-prescription system.

    With the exception of all but a handful of entries on the above list, almost all of these technologies are currently in use to some degree in the U.S. health care system. Drones are not yet widely used for medical deliveries; autonomous cars are only now being tested; and AI/machine learning and related technologies have not yet fully matured. But aside from these exceptions, it is impressive how many transformative technologies are already present—and in many instances, surprising that they have not yet come into broader use in health care.

Priority Issues for Advancing Technology Deployment and Development

The Technology Work Stream developed a list of high-priority issues for achieving a system of Health Care Without Walls. One set is focused on technology development; a second is focused on making broader use of technology and achieving a more distributed health care system through adopting and implementing technology; and a third set relates to the "infrastructure" (in the broadest sense) to support use of technology.

Technology Development Issues

As noted above, many technologies that will be deployed in the U.S. health care system in 2025 already exist, and to the degree they are in use at that time, they may well be employed more or less in the form in which they exist today. Still other technologies are under development and not yet in widespread use. The Technology Work Stream determined that it wanted to steer a list of recommendations to developers about how they should proceed to develop technologies that have a strong business case and that can deliver maximum usability. Technology Work Stream participants pointed to the fact that many start-ups lack a strong business plan or business case for their technology and may even gain Food and Drug Administration approval without having one. Often missing is any evidence base on the effects on cost and outcomes of a particular technology.

Verging into the area of human factors, work stream members also stressed that it would be important to avoid a repetition of what has occurred with the first generations of EHRs, which were developed largely on billing-related platforms; which have required large investments to customize them for users; and which are still not considered very usable by clinicians. They also expressed concerns about making sure that technologies are developed with patients in mind, particularly patients with low health literacy, cognitive issues, and other limitations.

To speed development of the most usable technologies, the Technology Work Stream recommends the following measures:

1. **There should be a serious nationwide effort to foster greater connections among entrepreneurs, technology developers, and clinicians to flesh out the Health Care Without Walls vision, and to articulate the most important**

challenges that clinicians, consumers, and payers face in adopting and using technology.

One approach that is being used in some health systems (such as Providence-St. Joseph, Inova, Bay State Health, and others) is to set up incubators inside their systems. These incubators enable start-up companies to team with clinicians who have expertise in the clinical process or business process, and engage in daily interaction. Such close cooperation could help prevent developers from creating solutions to "non-problems," or failing to fix problems that they do not know about, or that clinicians do not realize could be addressed. Another approach is for health systems to create or adopt university-style technology transfer process/advisory groups to help promising start-ups.

2. **Technology developers, and health system purchasers, should predicate all development and purchase of technology on the basis of total interoperability, seamless data and information exchange, high-quality data, and total data accessibility with appropriate privacy and security safeguards.**

Technologies should be easy to use and "frictionless" for users, seamlessly integrated into their lives so that they become an almost invisible part of the health care journey; transparent and allow those with more expertise to "interrogate" the system to examine the underlying digital coding and algorithms; interoperable, permitting exchange data exchange under open, common, and widely shared data standards. Data should follow the patient and be presented in such a way that they are clearly understood and actionable for users. Health systems, providers, and others should embrace a more collaborative open-source approach to sharing patient data (while preserving patient confidentiality) and exchange such data for the common good rather than hoard it for perceived competitive advantages.

3. **Develop specific partnerships between technology developers and small or safety-net health systems and critical-access hospitals.**

Some Technology Work Stream participants expressed the view that special steps should be taken to create technology development partnerships between technology developers and small or safety net health systems, which are unlikely to have the capabilities of larger systems to set up their own incubators and venture funds. A specific objective would be developing lower-cost technologies that would be affordable to these systems. One possibility would be to create federally or state-funded venture funds that would create this capacity for smaller systems. Through a competitive process, funding could be allocated to smaller health systems to incubate and test various innovations, somewhat analogous to the way the Innovation Center at the Centers for Medicare & Medicaid Services conducts various challenges to test innovative payment arrangements.

4. **Consider a range of human factors issues in technology development.**

Referring some issues to the Human Factors Work Stream for further discussion, the Technology Work Stream cited the following important considerations:

- Technologies should support team-based care and the clinician-patient relationship, along the lines of some of the principles adopted by the American Medical Association in 2016.[46] In particular, as the AMA principles state, technologies should "support care delivery that is patient-centered, promotes care coordination and facilitates team-based communication."

- Technologies should free up clinicians' time, so they can spend more time listening to patients and dealing with their problems.

- Technologies should make the health care experience more seamless for patients.[47]

- Technologies should improve work flow, particularly toward the goal of coordinating care.

- Technologies should be developed in such a way that they are usable for people with low health literacy or with cognitive difficulties. If not, the health care work force may need to be augmented to include individuals whose job will be to make certain that technologies are working for these types of patients. (For further information, see the Human Factors chapter of this report.)

- Technologies should be developed with a commitment to advancing health equity—the notion that everyone has a fair and just opportunity to be healthier, and that obstacles to health such as poverty, discrimination, and lack of access to education should be removed. Technological solutions must thus be based on data that are inclusive of underserved populations or those that are poor, lack access to education, optimal housing and other social and economic determinants of health and obstacles to greater health.

- Similarly, technologies should also be developed that can help health systems address the social and economic determinants of health and/or match patients to organizations and services that can help address their social needs. For example, analysis of EHRs that have been expanded to include a wealth of information from diverse sources (such as claims data from payers, patient data from providers and from patient questionnaires asking about social determinants, demographic data, environmental data, and other information) could help identify factors affecting the health of individuals and populations and point to useful interventions. Such information can be used to link patients with government programs and other resources such as housing, food banks, and utility reconnection services.

In a pilot project in Southern California, Kaiser Permanente partnered with a nonprofit organization called Health Leads to reach out to members in the Kaiser system who had been identified as being at highest risk of becoming "super-ultilizers" (in the top 1% of predicted utilization). Telephone screening by trained call-center workers revealed that 78 percent of those screened had at least one unmet social need, such as food insecurity or transportation issues; 74 percent of those with unmet needs agreed to enroll in the Health Leads program, which connects them with community resources such as food banks. By addressing many of the needs voiced by these respondents such as these, who preferred to be called "the Vital Few,"[48] Kaiser has kept patients from experiencing unnecessary visits and hospitalizations.[49]

Technology Procurement Issues

A major issue for all health systems will be making decisions about technology investment, particularly as care delivery models and the payment models that support them shift. The Technology Work Stream recognized that the Payment Work Stream would weigh in on this question, but also offered its own recommendations. The topic is complicated, as it is intimately tied up with the question of whether technologies will be reimbursed specifically, or whether health systems will need to invest in them without an expectation of reimbursement, at least initially or for some time to come.

An additional unknown is how quickly new payment models supporting technology-based activities such as telehealth will develop. Many payers have been reluctant to pay for telehealth for fear that doing so will simply drive up the number of virtual visits without displacing other forms of care (see Payment chapter of this volume for further discussion of this issue). If payment models develop widely to support use of technology and care displacement, health systems will have new incentives to acquire technology.

Separate and apart from its specific recommendations to the Payment Work Stream, the Technology Work Stream identified two recommendations for technology deployment:

1. **Create technology blueprints for health systems.**

    Given that some portion of technology purchases may ultimately not prove to have been wise investments, health systems could benefit from a thoughtful blueprint or toolkit guiding them through decisions about purchasing and using technologies. Although the private market of consultants and others may arise to meet this need, given the relatively thin margins of some hospitals and health systems, a publicly funded blueprint or toolkit could be valuable. There is precedent in other sectors for this kind of support, such as the U.S. Department of Agriculture's Cooperative Extension Service, or the regional extension services created by the HITECH provisions of the 2009 American Reinvestment and Recovery Act to foster the adoption of EHR's.

2. **Develop an evidence base and return-on-investment (ROI) analyses.**

    Given that many providers will want to minimize the risk of unwise investments, an evidence base demonstrating the cost effectiveness and cost-saving potential of technologies, as well as evidence about the effect of implementation of technologies on patient outcomes, is likely to be an important factor in promoting the adoption of such technologies.

Thus, for providers and payers to fully embrace a Health Care Without Walls system, more-distributed care must be cost-effective and achieve health outcomes for patients that are at least as equivalent to those achieved through traditional care delivery, and ideally superior to them. The issue is a complex one, in part because it's essential to consider not only the cost of implementing a technology and the infrastructure-related costs to maintaining it, but also system-level downstream costs.

For example, if a technology expands access to care, it might lead to increases in diagnostic testing and greater numbers of people diagnosed with conditions that require treatment. On the other hand, depending on the payment model (value-based care/accountable care models vs. fee for service), providing home-based services or other forms of support could save costs overall if it reduces unneeded care and errors or prevents illness or exacerbations of illnesses that require costly care, including hospital and emergency department visits. Thus, support is needed for studies that evaluate tech-enabled care and document its effects on costs and on patient outcomes. In addition, return-on-investment (ROI) studies should be conducted by a variety of organizations, private payers, health technology assessment organizations, and public agencies, including the Centers for Medicare & Medicaid, the Center for Medicare & Medicaid Innovation (the Innovation Center), the Agency for Healthcare Research and Quality, and others.

Infrastructure and Systems Issues to Support Technology Development and Use

The Technology Work Stream cited the importance of a number of "infrastructure" issues that must be addressed to support a more distributed, technology-enabled health care system. "Infrastructure" should be understood in its broadest possible context, as meaning the physical and organizational structures and facilities needed for operation of an enterprise.

Infrastructure also includes having the logistical capacity to deliver technologies where and when they are needed. For example, for "hospitalization at home" programs, one potential barrier might be difficulty getting a cart of equipment needed by a visiting clinician to a patient living in an apartment building lacking an elevator; ultimately, robotically assisted medial carts might provide a solution to scale stairs or navigate other difficult environmental features. Another aspect of logistics is being able to respond rapidly because of such factors as distance or traffic or road conditions. A hospital at home program offered by Presbyterian Healthcare Services in Albuquerque, New Mexico, requires a response time of two hours or less from vendors who deliver durable oxygen, durable medical equipment, intravenous medication, and diagnostic equipment such as mobile X-ray technology and ultrasound or electrocardiography equipment.

The state of the infrastructure supporting health information and information exchange will be especially critical. Work steam members identified several issues related to this issue:

1. **Address the issue of interoperability of health information and technology for fuller data and information exchange.**

    Interoperability is needed for continuous sharing of important care-related information and data among patients, providers, caregivers, payers, and organizations and for broad, secure collection and analysis of data (under suitable privacy and security protections). Achieving true interoperability would improve quality and continuity of care and patient safety, enhance data sharing through patient registries, support medical research, and provide incentives for innovators to create new products that could function in the health care information ecosphere.

    The problem of lack of interoperability should be understood at two levels. The first is the long-standing lack of sufficient interoperability of EHRs. The second is the absence of an infrastructure or set of protocols for exchanging broader sets of health information that originate outside of EHRs and are not protected health information under the federal Health Insurance Portability and Accountability Act (HIPAA) statute.

    Achieving EHR operability requires multiple steps. These measures include common data standards and a common communication language based on common vocabulary, structure, and format. Also needed is adoption of a proposed "trusted exchange framework," to advance a single "on-ramp" to interoperability. This set of public-private agreements would allow all types of health care stakeholders to join any health information network and to participate in nationwide exchange of health information, regardless of what health information technology developer they use, health information exchange or network they contract with, or where the patients' records are located.

In an ideal world, patient should have access to, and complete control, over their health care records, which can be stored for them in a trusted private repository personal health record or health record bank. Open application programming interfaces (APIs) are necessary to provide connections from personal health records to EHRs. (An open API is an interface available to all authorized users that can allow an application to send or receive data). EHR vendors have committed to making these open API's available to facilitate interoperability of EHR's, but progress has been slow.

`Furthermore, EHR vendors need to extend APIs to all of the significant data, including text documents, in the EHR and enable their EHRs to automatically update patient applications whenever the EHRs receive new data about the patient. Providers need to enable these APIs within their EHRs and make it easier for patients to connect their applications to these APIs. One simple change would be for providers to allow a patient to enter the address of his or her personal health record application into the patient portal of an E HR, so that the patient's application can be automatically copied on any new data received by the EHR.

As discussed further in the regulatory chapter of this volume, a number of other efforts are also under way within the federal and private sectors to advance initiatives addressing interoperability. Such initiatives as these need to proceed to fruition for health care without walls to become a reality. Also needed is a strategy for handling health-related patient data that originates from sources (such as remote sensors) that fall outside current laws and regulations. Currently, the federal Health Insurance Portability and Accountability Act (HIPAA), regulates the security of protected health information (PHI) in all mediums, including paper, electronic, and oral.

However, a growing amount of health information now being collected by devices such as remote sensors or exercise trackers falls outside of HIPAA's domain, and much of this information is expected to be integrated in EHRs and used in other ways. To protect the privacy and security of such data, it is essential that this issue be addressed to determine the best way forward, such an expansion of HIPAA rules or other regulatory action. (See the regulatory chapter for additional discussion of this issue).

2. **Achieve widespread access to fast, affordable broadband Internet.**

Fast and affordable broadband Internet access is crucial to achieving distributed health care and supporting public health outreach and education, especially for rural and remote areas. On the positive side, an estimated 77 percent of Americans currently subscribe to broadband Internet, and about 75 percent of rural households have broadband access. However, broadband is still unavailable or unaffordable to millions of Americans. (See further discussion of this issue in the Regulatory Work Stream chapter.)

One possible option to achieve worldwide access to high-speed broadband Internet, including to rural and remote areas, has been proposed by companies such as SpaceX, Google, OneWeb, Boeing, and Samsung. These companies have proposed a network of low-earth orbit satellites specifically for the purpose of expanded high speed Internet service in underserved locations around the world. SpaceX, for example, plans to launch more than 4,420 small low-orbit satellites in 2019, with full deployment expected by 2024, the company said in May 2017 testimony to the U.S. Senate. OneWeb Satellites, which is building a satellite factory at Kennedy Space Center's Exploration Park in Florida, is also currently building satellites in France for similar purposes.

As discussed more fully in the regulatory chapter of this volume, recent events in the regulatory sphere may complicate efforts to achieve broader access to universal and affordable high-speed broadband. The Federal Communications Commission decided in December 2017 to repeal the net neutrality regulations. These regulations prevented Internet service providers from raising costs for consumers or otherwise affecting broadband access, such as by blocking websites or charging for faster delivery of content to consumers.

There is great uncertainty about the impact of the repeal of net neutrality provisions, but of particular concern is the potential impact reduced Internet access would have on small and rural hospitals and providers. With the repeal of net neutrality, large Internet services providers could provide "fast lanes" for customers with more resources, such as large video-streaming services, and slow processing for those with modest resources. Telehealth services depend on the infrastructure of reliable and low-cost connectivity, and loss of net neutrality could undercut efforts to efforts to implement telehealth-related ventures, especially on small and rural hospitals and providers.[50] Additionally, IoT adoption could be affected by a loss of net neutrality, potentially creating situations where one proprietary IoT platform is granted access to high-speed "lanes" over another.

One additional and related issue that the work stream identified is the future of so-called Fifth Generation, or 5G, wireless cellular technology, which is estimated to deliver peak data download speeds about 100 times faster than the current standard, 4G, and will better enable such services as remote monitoring as devices connect directly to cellular towers. As 5G services is rolled out across the United States beginning this year, it remains to be seen how much and in what ways it may supplant broadband service, and how quickly it will come to areas of the country or individuals now facing challenges in access to broadband. The work stream recommended that this topic be monitored and potentially revisited over the next year and beyond.

3. **Ensure health information privacy and security.**

Patients, providers, and health systems need to have confidence in security and privacy protections for data generated and shared through various means, as well as assurance that medical devices are secure and protected against hacking. Failure to adequately protect patient data and security of devices can have such consequences as violations of HIPAA; identity theft; financial fraud; and other problems. Connectivity of devices in the "Internet of medical things" may result in digital eavesdropping and hacking of medical equipment.

For example, a ransomware attack that affected 48 hospitals in the United Kingdom in 2017 was enormously disruptive.[51] Access to medical records was blocked, and affected hospitals had to take MRI scanners and X-ray equipment offline and cancel medical procedures and appointments. In addition to privacy concerns, hacking of implanted medical devices has the potential to result in harm to patients. In August 2017, the FDA warned that 465,000 of certain models of pacemakers were vulnerable to hacking, and the agency advised that a firmware update (which providers could install noninvasively) had been created to fix the problem.

How the nation, and the world, should address security and privacy, especially with respect to the "Internet of medical things," is of paramount concern. Yet there is considerable uncertainty, ambiguity, and confusion about how this area might be regulated, which could impede development of a Health Care Without Walls ecosystem in many countries beyond the United

States. Policy recommendations, such a regulatory oversight, to address this issue are set forth in the regulatory chapter of this volume.

In addition to these and other regulatory issues, developers of digital devices and systems must consider what technological tools can be brought to bear to ensure privacy and security of health information, including appropriate de-identification of health data collected for the purpose of analyzing population health trends. For example, blockchain technology may be useful in enhancing data security.

4. **Continued development of the evidence base on the effects of digital technologies on cost and outcomes**

    Because new technologies arise, and older ones improve and evolve, ongoing research to study cost-effectiveness and effects on outcomes is a necessary component of the infrastructure of a technology-enabled Health Care Without Walls system.

5. **Explore and promote payment models that support distributed care**

    Because fee-for-service payment will remain a barrier to adoption of many technologies, work stream members noted that building the case to move to a value-based payment system will be important for a Health Care Without Walls system to evolve and flourish. Total cost will need to be budget neutral, so initiatives that document long-term cost savings are essential. For example, providing home-based services and other forms of support could save costs overall if it ultimately curbs unneeded care, prevents illness or exacerbations of illness that require costly care, and reduces hospital and emergency department visits.

Summary Recommendations

In sum, the Technology Work Stream identified a number of issues that need to be addressed to support optimal development of digital health technologies, foster their deployment, and ensure the necessary infrastructure to support them, to realize the vision of Health Care Without Walls.

Recommendations for technology development

1. **There should be a serious nationwide effort to connect entrepreneurs, technology developers, and technologists with clinicians, patients, and policy makers to expand on the Health Care Without Walls vision, and to articulate the most important challenges that clinicians, consumers, and payers face in adopting and using technology. The federal government could lead the way, in partnership with states and leading health care organizations.**

    Entrepreneurs and technologists need to identify the problems that are most meaningful for clinicians and patients and understand the most important challenges that clinicians, consumers, and payers face in using technology. To ensure that such awareness and understanding exists, it is essential to bring technology developers together with clinicians, so they have ongoing contact with each other.

    Larger health systems should be encouraged to set up in-house incubators to ensure the kind of daily interactions that will promote mutual recognition of the problems that clinicians and patients face, and that could be alleviated or mitigated by adoption of innovative technology. Health systems should also be encouraged to create or adopt a university-style technology transfer process and/or assemble advisory groups to help promising start-ups develop innovative products or services.

2. **The federal government should provide seed money for small or safety-net systems and rural hospitals to develop new prototypes of technology-enabled, distributed care suitable in their settings.**

    Small or safety-net systems, and rural facilities such as critical-access hospitals, need to be part of the process of developing technology that not only supports a more distributed health care system in general, but also promotes the development of lower-cost technologies that these systems could afford. Technology Work Stream participants suggest that the creation of federally or state-funded venture funds could provide innovation funding for technology-enabled care for smaller groups, who are unlikely to have the resources to set up their own incubators or venture funds. Government funders could allocate support through a competitive process to smaller health systems to incubate and test innovation.

3. **Technology innovators should take a range of health care and human factors into account and address them as they create and adapt technologies to enable more distributed care.**

   Technology Work Stream members cited a range of human factors issues that should be components of digital technologies. These include supporting team-based care and the clinician-patient relationship; freeing up clinicians' time so they can spend more time with patients, particularly those with complex health issues; making the health care experience more seamless for patients; improving work flow and promoting coordination of care; striving to develop technologies that can be used by people with low health literacy or cognitive difficulties; and incorporating elements that help health systems address social and economic determinants of health. (For a more complete discussion of these issue, see the Human Factors chapter of this volume.)

4. **More effective early-stage assessments.**

   At an early stage of development, technology developers need to understand the proper audience or customer base for a product (consumer vs professional) and consider the net (downstream) costs of implementing it.

5. **Help decision makers and health systems prioritize technologies with a blueprint or toolkit.**

   Health systems, especially those with relatively thin margins, face challenges in making decisions about technology investment. A publicly funded blueprint or toolkit could be a valuable asset to provide guidance about acquiring and implementing technologies.

6. **Develop an evidence base.**

   Steps should be taken to develop an evidence base on the cost-effectiveness of technologies and the effects of technologies on patient outcomes. Particular attention should be paid to ensuring that evidence is developed that pertains to the effectiveness of technologies in meeting the needs of underserved populations.

7. **Develop strategies to reach special populations.**

    Strategies are needed to help educate uninsured/underinsured people, and/or people with low literacy/health literacy, about the digital health care services that are or will be available to them. Particular attention also should be paid to ensuring that underserved populations can gain access to, and use of, these technologies and services.

Recommendations for technology infrastructure

1. **Ensure interoperability of the technology of health care.** Promote international standards on transmission of health care data through standard document formats and open APIs. Stay abreast of consensus on and promote semantic-interoperability standards that allow patient data from the sending EHR to be used effortlessly by a provider seeing the patient using the receiving EHR. Insist that all EHRs have a place to store the address of the patient's personal health record so that patient can sign up once with each of their providers and then automatically receive a complete copy of their health record and any new data that arrive at that facility without further effort.

2. **Achieve nationwide broadband or satellite-enabled Internet access.** See recommendations in the Regulatory chapter of this volume.

3. **Focus on privacy and security.** Support efforts to assure privacy protections and security of patient data generated and shared in telehealth and other areas (including appropriate de-identification of health data collected for the purpose of analyzing population health trends), as well as protect against hacking of devices. (See regulatory chapter for further recommendations.)

Technology and Health Care Without Walls: Chapter 1 in Brief

1. The Information Age and digital revolution have given rise to a host of technologies that are enabling the evolution of "distributed" health care outside of conventional institutional settings. Many of these technologies are described in the "Glossary" section of this chapter of the report. Because of these technologies, it is increasingly possible to contemplate what were once seemingly futuristic scenarios—such as an elderly patient with a heart condition being monitored remotely, alerted by his health care providers in the event they detect an issue with his heart rate, and dispatching an

autonomous (driverless) "medi-car" outfitted with medical sensors and other testing and communication devices to further assess his condition.

2. The beginnings of this technological transformation of health care are already evident in the home and in other settings. Technologies such as wearable sensors and smart phones, along with capabilities such as artificial intelligence, machine learning, and advanced data analytics, hold the promise of more effective ways to support individuals in preserving their health, as well as to predict, diagnose, and treat disease, enabled by collection of personalized data (from wearable sensors, smart phones, genomics, and other data sources) and the use of artificial intelligence, machine learning, and data analytics.

3. All of these technologies, including digital tools and new channels for delivering health care services in a system built on "Health Care Without Walls" concepts, offer potentially large benefits to individuals and to the nation. Put simply, the vision within reach is of a health care system that is far more accessible and convenient, improves quality of care, removes some of the friction in health care, makes better use of clinicians, improves care coordination, "democratizes" care through the spread of knowledge and expertise, facilitates public health and population health strategies, potentially lowers the cost of care, and offers a host of other benefits as well.

4. The Technology Work Stream of the Health Care Without Walls initiative was charged with examining current and future technologies that could realistically be in place, and widely used, in the U.S. health care system in 2025, assuming that barriers to their adoption were addressed. The work stream crafted a vision of the future through a set of scenarios depicting care options for various patients and populations, and detailing how care could be delivered to them with the aid of an array of technologies. It also helped to identify barriers to deployment and take-up of technologies, in conjunction with the other work streams, and drafted recommendations for changes in public policy and within health care organizations, payers, and others, to support the 2025 technology vision and stimulate advocacy to achieve this vision.

5. The Technology Work Stream concluded that technologies used in the delivery of Health Care Without Walls should have common elements and key features, including usability across many different types of patients and providers; transparency as to the underlying digital coding and algorithms of

any technology, so that any biases or other limitations can be detected; interoperability; a commitment to data sharing and information and exchange, albeit within a framework that enhances data privacy and security; and seamless connectivity with other technologies. These technologies should be able to depend upon universal internet and affordable high-speed broadband access nationwide.

6. The Technology Work Stream noted numerous challenges to the adoption of technology, including those that will be discussed in subsequent chapters around payment, regulation, and the work force. Beyond these, which will be discussed at length, it noted that the history of adoption of information technology in health care is riddled with examples of hugely expensive projects gone awry. In particular, the adoption of electronic health records technology has been plagued by huge costs, a perceived lack of usability, and failure to achieve system-wide interoperability. It will be critical to avoid the mistakes of the past as new technologies are adopted into health care.

7. The work stream made a series of recommendations about how to advance Health Care Without Walls from a technological standpoint.

8. First and foremost, there should be a serious nationwide effort to foster greater connections among entrepreneurs, technology developers, and clinicians to flesh out the Health Care Without Walls vision, and to articulate the most important challenges that clinicians, consumers, and payers face in adopting and using technology. The federal government could lead the way, in partnership with states, technology companies, and leading health care organizations.

9. A blueprint or toolkit should be created, perhaps through a public-private initiative, to provide guidance to health care organizations and systems about acquiring and implementing technologies to enable more virtual and distributed care. An evidence base should be created and disseminated on the cost-effectiveness of technologies and the effects on patient outcomes and costs.

10. Partnerships should be created between technology developers and small or safety-net health systems and critical-access hospitals to develop and/or adapt technologies to their specific needs and cost structures. The federal government should provide seed money for small or safety-net systems and

rural hospitals to develop new prototypes of technology-enabled, distributed care suitable in their settings.

11. Technology developers, and health system purchasers, should predicate all development and purchase of technology on the basis of total interoperability, seamless data and information exchange, high-quality data, and total data accessibility with appropriate privacy and security safeguards.

12. Technology innovators should take a range of health care and human factors into account and address them as they create and adapt technologies to enable more distributed care. These include supporting team-based care and the clinician-patient relationship; freeing up clinicians' time so they can spend more time with patients, particularly those with complex health issues; making the health care experience more seamless for patients; improving clinical work flow; and promoting the coordination of care. In addition to thinking through how technologies can best address such issues, technology developers at any early stage of their work must understand the proper audience or customer base for a product, and consider the net downstream costs of implementing it.

13. Technologies should be developed in such a way that they are usable for people with low health literacy, cognitive difficulties, and other physical and mental disabilities. Strategies should be developed to help reach **and** educate uninsured/underinsured people, and/or people with low literacy/health literacy, about the digital health care services that are or will be available to them.

14. Technologies should be developed with a commitment to advancing health equity—the notion that everyone has a fair and just opportunity to be healthier, and that obstacles to health such as poverty, discrimination, and lack of access to education should be removed. Technological solutions must thus be based on data that are inclusive of underserved populations or those that are poor, lack access to education, optimal housing and other social and economic determinants of health and obstacles to greater health.

15. Technologies should also be developed that can help health systems address the social and economic determinants of health and/or match patients to organizations and services that can help address their social needs. For example, analysis of EHRs that have been expanded to include a wealth of information from diverse sources (such as claims data from payers, patient

data from providers and from patient questionnaires asking about social determinants, demographic data, environmental data, and other information) could help identify factors affecting the health of individuals and populations and point to useful interventions. Such information can be used to link patients with government programs and other resources such as housing, food banks, and utility reconnection services.

◆ ◆ ◆

End Notes, Chapter 1

[29] Keith Montgomery, "Kaiser Center for Total Health," filmed May 10, 2017 at Health Care Without Walls Convening, video, https://www.youtube.com/watch?v=FQ21OIuGgUM&list=PLaB2YSdeiN4W743cwOVErm_CoFw_AJYj6&index=2.

[30] Eric Topol, *The Patient Will See You Now: The Future of Medicine is in Your Hands* (New York: Basic Books, 2015).

[31] Kurt Mattson, "The Digital Pill Presents Privacy Issues," Forensis Group (January 2018), https://www.forensisgroup.com/digital-pill-presents-privacy-issues/.

[32] See https://www.pwc.com/gx/en/issues/analytics/assets/pwc-ai-analysis-sizing-the-prize-report.pdf.

[33] Nic Fleming, "How artificial intelligence is changing drug discovery," *International journal of science* 557, (2018): S55-S57, DOI: 10.1038/d41586-018-05267-x.

[34] See https://www.healthit.gov/sites/default/files/jsr-17-task-002_aiforhealthandhealthcare12122017.pdf.

[35] Saurabh Jha et al., "Adapting to Artificial Intelligence," *JAMA* 316, no. 22 (December 2016): 2353-2354. DOI: 10.1001/jama.2016.17438.

[36] See https://cancer.osu.edu/blog/james-team-breaks-new-ground-with-digital-pathology-cancer-diagnosis.

[37] "UMMC 2 You," University of Mississippi Medical Center Health Care, https://www.umc.edu/Healthcare/Telehealth/UMMC%202%20You/UMMC%202%20You.html.

[38] Sharad Manaktala, "Evaluating the Impact of a Computerized Surveillance Algorithm and Decision Support System on Sepsis Mortality" *Journal of the American Medical Informatics Assoication* 24, no. 1 (January 2017): 88-95, https://doi.org/10.1093/jamia/ocw056.

[39] See https://www.pwc.com/gx/en/issues/analytics/assets/pwc-ai-analysis-sizing-the-prize-report.pdf.

[40] David Lazer et al., "The Parable of Google Flu: Traps in Big Data Analysis," *Science Magazine* 343, no. 6176 (March 2014): 1203-1205, DOI: 10.1126/science.1248506.

[41] David Lazer et al., "What We Can Learn From the Epic Failure of Google Flu Trends," Wired (October 2015), https://www.wired.com/2015/10/can-learn-epic-failure-google-flu-trends/.

[42] VHA Telehealth Services, "VHA Telehealth Quarterly Newsletter," (January 2016), https://www.telehealth.va.gov/newsletter/2016/Newsletter_Vol15Iss01.pdf.

[43] Alex D. Federman et al., "Association of a Bundled Hospital-at-Home and 30-Day Postacute Transitional Care Program with Clinical Outcomes and Patient Experiences," *JAMA internal medicine*, (2018), DOI: 10.1001/jamainternmed.2018.2562.

[44] "How it Works," Big White Wall, accessed April 1, 2017, https://www.bigwhitewall.com/V2/about.aspx.

[45] Michael Poku et al., "Patient Relationship Management: What the US Healthcare System can Learn from Other Industries," *JGIM*, (August 2016), DOI: 10.1007/s11606-016-3836-6.

[46] See, https://www.ama-assn.org/ama-adopts-principles-promote-safe-effective-mhealth-applications.

[47] Paula Braveman et al., "What is Health Equity?" Report by University of California San Francisco and Robert Wood Johnson Foundation, May 2017, www.rwjf.org/content/dam/farm/reports/issue_briefs/2017/rwjf437393.

[48] Verbal communication, Nirav Shah, then of Kaiser Permanente, in 2017.

[49] Nirav Shah, "Health Care that Targets Unmet Social Needs," NEJM Catalyst, April 13, 2016, https://catalyst.nejm.org/health-care-that-targets-unmet-social-needs/.

[50] Meg Bryant, "Loss of Net Neutrality Could Slow Telehealth Access," Healthcare Dive, January 11, 2018, https://www.healthcaredive.com/news/net-neutrality-healthcare-telehealth/514018/.

[51] Damien Gayle et al., "NHS Seeks to Recover from Global Cyber-Attack as Security Concerns Resurface" The Guardian, May 13, 2017, https://www.theguardian.com/society/2017/may/12/hospitals-across-england-hit-by-large-scale-cyber-attack.

SCENARIO 3: A TEEN WITH DIABETES AND FATHER WITH CONGESTIVE HEART FAILURE STAY AT HOME WITH THEIR CONDITIONS CONTROLLED

MICHAEL, 17, is a U.S.-born son of legal immigrants (now naturalized U.S. citizens) who lives with his family in an exurban area outside a major Eastern U.S. city. He has Type I diabetes and is insulin dependent; he also has some mental health issues—a combination of mild depression and obsessive-compulsive disorder.

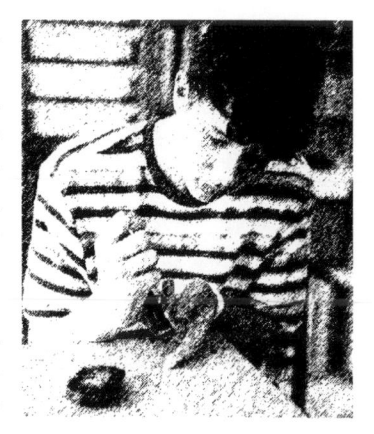

Michael's father, George, is 48, and disabled with congestive heart failure. Michael's mother, Mary, works as a home-health aide and is the family breadwinner. She is mostly healthy, but she also works long hours, and suffers stress due to her role as main caregiver for husband and son. Between the mother's income and the father's disability support, the family is struggling to stay afloat.

Approximately 1.25 million U.S. children and adults have type 1 diabetes like Michael, and in youth under age 20, about 17,900 are diagnosed with diabetes annually. (A total population of 30.3 million Americans is estimated to have both diagnosed and undiagnosed diabetes.) Diabetes is officially deemed the 7th leading cause of death in the United States. People with diabetes are also at greater risk of depression.

For these diabetes sufferers, as for Michael, the key goals are much the same: maintain adequate control of the diabetes, avert complications, and enable them to stay as healthy as possible. It's also especially vital to treat Michael's mental health issues appropriately. Michael wants to finish high school and attend community college, and eventually get a good job to advance his and his family's economic circumstances.

For Michael's father, George, the goals are similar: treat his congestive heart failure, and help him maintain a healthy diet and avoid weight gain. George has had several emergency hospitalizations in the past several years due to the heart failure. Since, as a disabled person, he has qualified for Medicare, hospitals are now penalized if he and other patients experience too many avoidable readmissions within 30 days of discharge.

As Michael was born and raised in the United States, his English is fluent, but his parents' English is still halting, and they mostly speak their native language at home. Like many residents of the United States with relatively low proficiency in English, the parents also have low rates of health literacy. In the past, these issues have posed problems for the family. When Michael was first diagnosed with Type 1 diabetes several years ago, no medical interpreter was present when clinicians conveyed the news, and as a result, the parents didn't really understand the gravity of Michael's condition and the importance of keeping his blood glucose levels under control. On occasion, Michael developed the standard symptoms of hypoglycemia— rapid heartbeat, pale skin, numbness, and slurred speech—and had to be rushed to the emergency department for care.

Today, Michael is on Medicaid, and his care is organized and financed through a Medicaid managed care organization that is unusually proactive about both care coordination through a "medical home" model, and about deploying technologies to assist patients in staying healthy and in the community. It equips Michael, first, with a clinical case manager/navigator who is very technology savvy, and also expert at helping younger people manage their chronic conditions. He coordinates the process through which Michael obtains a smart continuous glucose monitor and automated insulin pump. The smart CGM provides glucose readings every five minutes, reducing the need for fingerstick tests; it sends information about Michael's readings automatically to the insulin pump, which adjusts Michael's insulin accordingly. It also sends information to Michael's clinical care team and, via an app, to Michael's mother, so that she can stay on top of his situation as well. On Michael's care team are his endocrinologist, a primary care physician, a certified diabetes educator, and a clinical pharmacist, who not only often participate as a team in telehealth "visits" with Michael, but also meet virtually as a group to discuss his case.

To help Michael with his mental health issues, the managed care organization has also connected Michael with a psychiatrist, a psychopharmacologist, and a mental health nurse, who hold regular telehealth visits with Michael and with the rest of the care team. They've prescribed an antidepressant for Michael, and also introduced Michael to a service with a smart app that draws on cognitive behavioral therapy approaches to help him manage his depression and OCD. A community health worker also stops by Michael's home, or has FaceTime visits with Michael, to check on him and his conditions. She has also introduced Michael to a psychiatric social worker on the team, who is stepping in to serve as a "life coach" to Michael as he prepares to finish high school and head to college.

George, Michael's father, struggled with his condition before he became eligible for Medicare, but now he is enrolled in a Medicare Advantage Special Needs Plan (SNP) that is also proactive on the technology front, operates on a "medical home" model, and is committed to helping George stay healthy and at home. George's care, like Michael's, is coordinated by case manager. On George's care team are both a cardiologist and a primary care physician, who meet with him regularly via telehealth; a professional medical interpreter also participates to assist with any language issues. He has a digital scale in his home that he uses to weigh himself regularly, as well as an app that conducts electrocardiograms from his smart phone; the results are transmitted directly to his care team. The SNP plan also provides transportation as needed to any medical appointments.

A nutritionist on the team also consults with George regularly via telehealth, and has taught him to use an app and scanner that can help him analyze the nutritional content of the foods he eats. Another community health worker employed by the plan visits regularly; he is bilingual, and from the same ethnic group as George, and has become a vital source of connection between George and his care team. As a result, George has now gone almost a full year without an exacerbation of his condition that requires an emergency department visit or a hospitalization.

Finally, in a highly atypical arrangement, the Medicaid managed care organization and the Medicare Advantage Special Needs Plan have adopted a "family connections" policy, in which they attempt to link the case managers of chronically ill relatives in the same family. Both Michael and George have authorized their case managers to meet virtually several times a year and discuss their cases, and their family's situation, jointly. Through one of these consultations, the case managers learned that Mary, Michael's mother and George's wife, was suffering from chronic stress and was herself in need of support. They were able to connect her with a community wellness program that focuses on meditation and yoga, and that offered a peer support group for individuals coping with family illness.

Now, with everyone's health stabilized, the family is looking forward to celebrating Michael's high school graduation, and excited that he'll begin his two years of tuition-free community college soon.

◆ ◆ ◆

SCENARIO 4: A CHRONICALLY ILL COUPLE IN A RURAL AREA

JOE IS A 52-year-old male who lives in a rural area of a state in the upper Midwest. He is jobless, having lost a job several years ago running a forklift at a now-defunct small manufacturing plant, and having been unable to find suitable reemployment. In the meantime, he developed chronic back pain, and is now on disability. He takes Oxycontin to relieve the pain. As a former smoker, Joe also has chronic obstructive pulmonary disease, as well as depression.

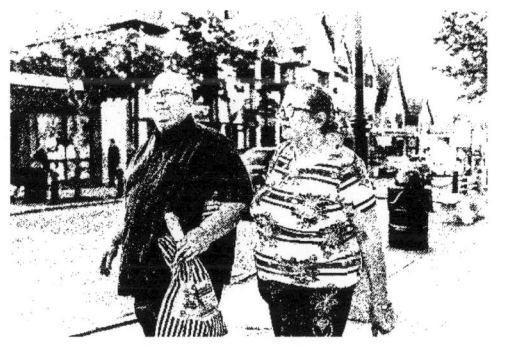

Ann, Joe's wife, is 51, and has worked for years at the cash register of a local convenience store. She is obese, and has both hypertension and Type II diabetes. The area in which Joe and Ann live has few amenities conducive to maintaining optimal health. It qualifies as a "food desert" because nearest full-line supermarket is nearly 90 minutes away by car. The nearest critical access hospital is 12 miles from their home. The couple receives medical care from one of area's few primary care physicians, but are currently not receiving care from any specialists. Joe and Ann have one car, and no internet access at home since they can't afford it. High-speed broadband internet access has not yet come to their part of the state.

Because of his disability, Joe is now covered by Medicare, and Ann has qualified for Medicaid under the state's recent expansion of the program. The couple's two children moved away years ago, and now live in cities that are several states away.

Joe and Ann are far from alone in their battles with chronic illness. Low back pain is the single leading cause of disability worldwide, according to the Global Burden of Disease Study, and the second most common cause of disability in U.S. adults. Almost 15.7 million Americans report that they have been diagnosed with chronic lower respiratory disease, primarily COPD, which was the third leading cause of death in the United States in 2014. Of the 20.5 million Americans 12 or older that had a substance use disorder in 2015, 2 million had a substance use disorder involving prescription pain relievers such as Oxycontin. An estimated 30 million Americans have diabetes. Almost 40 percent of U.S. adults, or approximately 98 million people, are obese.

Joe's and Ann's rural location, and the paucity of health care providers and services in their area, make it hard to achieve what would be considered optimal care goals. Joe would be well served if he could be eased off the Oxycontin, perhaps with a prescription for suboxone, and try other non-opioid approaches to pain relief, including physical therapy. His COPD and depression need to be treated appropriately; more than once, an exacerbation of the COPD led him to be rushed to the critical access hospital for several-day stays. It's not out of the realm of possibility that Joe's health could be restored to such a level that he, too, could resume working, at least part-time. As for Ann, she would benefit from at least a modest amount of weight loss and avoidance of any further weight gain, and appropriate medication and lifestyle interventions to keep her hypertension and Type 2 diabetes under control. She has had occasional instances of hypoglycemia that have also resulted in admissions to the critical access hospital.

Fortunately for Joe and Ann, the governor and legislature of their state have taken a highly proactive approach, and encouraged the state's Medicaid program, as well as Medicare Advantage plans operating in the state, to form relationships with the one large academic medical center in the state capital, several hundred miles away from where Joe and Ann live. The result has been transformational.

First, both the Medicaid managed care organization in which Ann is enrolled, and Joe's Medicare Advantage plan, gave the couple their first smart phones. (There is now cellular service in their area, and satellite internet service is scheduled to arrive in about a year). Now, they have Facetime visits with their care coordinators at their health plans, as well as with physicians and nurse practitioners from the academic medical center. Joe has consulted with a specialist in opioid use disorder, who prescribed suboxone for him; he also was paired with a physical therapist, who came to Joe's home to train him on simple exercises for his back, and now checks in regularly via FaceTime. Joe also now has a wearable device that monitors his physical activity and pain, and send data to his clinical team at the academic medical center so they can stay informed and consult back with Joe as needed. He also has access to telehealth visits with a behavioral health care provider to help treat his depression, and was connected with an app that employs cognitive behavioral therapy approaches to assist in a form of self-care.

Meanwhile, under a special grant from Congress, transformation of the role of the critical access hospital is under way. The hospital is now converting to be a community health care "hub" that will offer telemedicine consultations with the academic medical center, and a small observation unit for local residents who are sick and may need to be hospitalized. A new emergency transportation system is being developed to transport very ill people from the state's rural areas to the academic medical center as needed. Autonomous cars are scheduled for arrival in the area by 2025, and will be a further means of addressing local transportation needs.

A small local corps of community health providers has been trained and now operate out of the "community health hub" in the former critical access hospital. They visit Joe and Ann regularly. One community health care worker took Ann shopping to show her what foods she should purchase and eat to help control her diabetes. The community health worker also advised regularly walking, and showed Ann how to use an app on her phone that can help her track her diet and her physical activity. Ann's Medicaid managed care organization also pioneered in delivering a virtual version of the Diabetes Prevention Program, which Ann participated in via cell phone.

On both Joe's and Ann's care teams are pharmacists, who check in regularly via FaceTime with Joe and Ann about their medications. They have linked with the one community pharmacist in the Joe's and Ann's area, and coordinate dispensing of prescriptions. For now, the community health workers can pick up prescriptions and take them to Joe and Ann, but with online retailers now developing pharmacy operations, it's likely that such services may ultimately be the way Joe and Ann obtain their medications. Similarly, Ann's Medicaid managed care organization is now planning to begin paying for delivery of healthy foods by a national online food service as a way of helping Ann control her diabetes.

A year after the launch of these new programs, Joe and Ann are practically different people. Joe no longer takes Oxycontin, experiences far less back pain, his COPD is under control, and his depression has lifted. Ann has dropped 10 pounds and is committed to losing more. The couple's diet now focuses on more healthful foods and smaller portions; they take long walks together in the evenings, when Ann gets home from work. They've formed strong bonds with the community health workers, as well as their providers from the academic medical center, whom they've never met in person but who they consider part of their community. They're now planning a trip to visit their children and grandchildren in those seemingly far-away cities—a first.

◆ ◆ ◆

CHAPTER 2: PAYMENT AND REIMBURSEMENT TO SUPPORT HEALTH CARE WITHOUT WALLS

THE ROLE OF economic incentives— i.e., payment and reimbursement of health care providers, as well as other actors in the system—is critically important in health care, especially for the largest and costliest system in the world: that of the United States. How, then, will payment and reimbursement policies within health care support the movement toward more distributed forms of health care, more focus on the upstream drivers of health status, and adoption and use of a broad range of technologies in the new delivery platform?

The Payment and Reimbursement Work Stream of the Health Care Without Walls initiative considered which payment models would best support these more distributed forms of health care, while also linking payment to improved patient outcomes, greater efficiency, and better overall value for the dollars expended. During the course of its discussions, the work stream had six major goals, as follows:

1) Taking into account the vision developed by the Technology Work Stream, define what payment models and reimbursement arrangements will best support a vision of more distributed care in 2025;

2) Define payment and reimbursement models that will support interventions and activities to improve the health of all Americans, not just to supply care to those already sick; and in particular, to advance the health of those within the population whose underlying health status is most likely to be jeopardized by low incomes and levels of education, lack of economic opportunity, lack of access to healthful food and housing, and other ingredients of a healthy life.

3) Recognizing the transition under way by many providers from fee-for-service care to new payment models, including Advanced Alternative Payment Models under the Medicare Quality Payment Program.[52] identify features of reimbursement and payment that will support the Health Care Without Walls vision while also enabling and reinforcing the movement to AAPMs;

4) Draft a set of recommendations for changes in public policy and by health care organizations, payers, and others, to support the 2025 Health Care Without Walls vision;

5) Pose issues that other work streams should tackle and/or recommendations that they should make to support the transition to new payment models that allow for more distributed care;

6) Identify any critical research gaps about new payment models that must be filled as the nation moves to a more flexible health care system.

The points of departure for the Payment and Reimbursement Work Stream were first, to consider the range of technologies that will underpin the evolving distributed health care system; and second, to consider the current state of payment, particularly with respect to the use of technologies and the provision of various forms of distributed health care outside of conventional institutional settings. An overview of both appears below.

Following this examination of the current state of payment and technology, the work stream undertook a third step: Describing and articulating a new payment paradigm that would drive innovation toward more distributed, technology-enabled forms of care, rather than merely accommodating some technological innovation, as the payment system does now, or paying directly for specific technologies. These recommendations are laid out in the final portion of this chapter.

The Current Payment & Reimbursement Landscape and How It Accommodates Technologies

As noted in the Technology Work Stream chapter of this report, when Health Care Without Walls refers to "technologies," it includes information technologies that gather and/or transmit data and information, or that use digital information in novel ways. Technology is therefore considered in the broadest sense, to include items that are conventionally deemed technology—such as robotics or smart devices—as well as the entire digital universe of artificial or augmented intelligence, cognitive computing, and information analytics. The current payment system in health care accommodates these and other technologies in a variety of ways, as discussed below.

How Technology is Paid For in Health Care: Overview

Payment in the U.S. health care system is complex, highly fragmented, decentralized, open to fraud, and both confusing and confounding to providers, payers, and the public. It is still largely based on payment per unit of service, resulting in total payment that grows with the volume of care delivered. U.S. payment systems only recently have been linked more closely to value, often measured by intermediate indicators (e.g., blood glucose level test results for diabetes patients) or other proxies for outcomes that measure real improvements in the lives of patients. A full discussion of the multiple dimensions of payment in U.S. health care is beyond the scope of this paper, but it has been widely argued that current payment methodologies, by driving volume, have played an important role in rising overall outlays for medical goods and services in the United States. The transition to new forms of payment, resulting from the effort to extract more value out of the system than volume, is discussed more fully below.

Technology in the U.S. health care system is paid for in especially complicated and variable ways. When hospitals, physician offices, and other health care providers purchase new technology, these purchases are typically considered capital expenditures, as they would be with any other business. The cost of these investments is amortized or depreciated over time, and big purchases are often financed through debt, or borrowing. In this respect, the payment system finances much of the technology in health care indirectly, in that payment for services to providers yields revenue that can be used at least in part to pay for capital investments that are depreciated over time.

Generally speaking, the payment and reimbursement policies of both public and private sector payers (insurers and employers) do not <u>directly</u> pay for technology acquisition and use. Rather, payment is generally set to pay for services that a physician or other health care provider delivers to a patient. Technology is paid for indirectly, as a recognized cost input into the provision of care. For example, a clinician might be paid for administering and interpreting an X-ray; this payment in effect pays indirectly, but not directly, for the use of the X-ray machine. Similarly, the payment system will not pay directly for the cost of purchasing a surgical robot, but it will compensate the surgeon for performing the surgery delivered with the aid of the robot. The technology's cost is accounted for within the payment that is established or agreed upon for the particular payment code accounting for that service.

A key question is always this one: When is the use of technology part of a core service that is already being delivered and paid for, and when does it constitute an entirely new or different service that should be paid for separately? This question may grow somewhat complicated in an era in which technology is advancing and the way that services are delivered is changing.

On the hospital inpatient side in Medicare, the Centers for Medicare and Medicaid Services (CMS) can update its prospective payment rates to hospitals over time to accommodate the use of new technologies. However, there is typically in these updates, as new technologies must first be in use for some time, and their costs also must be reflected in the data CMS uses to set payment rates. Furthermore, payment rates are adjusted across services in a way that does not increase the federal budget deficit, so there is no net overall increase in payment.

Medicare also has a separate provision, known as "new technology add-on payments," (NTAPs), which were created to recognize the costs of new medical technologies as they are incorporated into existing services, and before CMS has had a chance to update prospective payment rates to accommodate the technological change. However, these payments are limited to specific, extraordinarily expensive treatments, and typically do not cover the full costs of acquiring or administering them.

Another way in which technology costs are incorporated into payment for health care is through the Medicare Physician Payment Fee Schedule. The fee schedule relies on national "relative value units," or RVU's, that rank on a common scale the resources used to provide medical services, such as the physician's work, the expenses of the physician's practice, and the costs of professional liability (malpractice) insurance. All of these factors are adjusted for geographic cost variations, and multiplied by a so-called conversion factor (to convert the RVUs into payment rates). When a new technology is developed that may be implemented into the provision of a service, resulting in a higher quality of that service, the cost of this technology is considered in the practice expense component of the payment calculation. In this way, the cost of the technology is attributed to a service in payment for that service.

RVU's are calculated in part based on the input of the American Medical Association/Specialty Society RVS Update Committee, or RUC, which advises CMS in developing them. But it typically takes time for the RUC to review the expenses, technological or otherwise, that are associated with the provision of a service, and to make any recommendation as to technological or other developments that need to be accounted for in the valuation of the service. Thus, there can be a lag in the process through which the costs of technology are factored into payment.

Because of this gap between the speed at which technology develops, and the speed at which the system compensates clinicians for the use of that technology, providers aren't always motivated to adopt new technologies quickly. Lagged updates in payment simply don't allow them to realize a return on, or even amortize, the technology investment in a short period of time. Other than through the slow development of updates to the relative value units associated with Current Procedural Terminology (CPT) codes—the codes used to report medical, surgical, and diagnostic procedures and services to entities such as physicians, health insurance companies, and accreditation organizations – there is only modest payment support for the capital expenditures for doctors' offices, hospitals, or other providers (with the notable exception of durable medical equipment, as discussed below).

Providers' motivation, then, to buy and integrate new technology is often simply to enhance and improve patient care, or to reduce effort or the costs of production (whether or not the evidence supports these suppositions, as will be discussed further below). But the payment implications of new technologies are a serious consideration for providers who are considering acquiring them, and these may militate against investments in technology until the costs are incorporated into updated payment amounts.

Public Payers: Past Precedents in Restraining or Stimulating Technology Use in Health Care

Government and public payers also influence the acquisition of technology by health care providers. Three examples relevant to the Health Care Without Walls initiative illustrate this reality and yield important lessons: (1) the "certificate of need" programs instituted in the 1960s and '70s; (2) efforts to create a national interoperable network of electronic health records over the past two decades; and (3) the establishment of a competitive bidding program for durable medical equipment in the 2000s.

Certificate of Need: With hospital construction and costs escalating beyond forecasts, states began to experiment with certificate of need (CON) laws in the 1960s. These laws aimed to restrain the construction of unnecessary hospitals and nursing homes, but also the purchase of duplicative, costly technologies such as imaging machines within a defined geographic area.

The Health Planning Resources Development Act, adopted by the U.S. Congress and signed into law in 1974, propelled CON forward significantly. The law required all 50 states to have health planning agencies to evaluate and grant approvals to hospitals for major capital projects and expenditures. Federal money was allocated to fund the initiative. By 1978, 36 states had CON laws, and by the mid-1980s, all states except Louisiana had a CON law. States were variably active in enforcing these statutes, but many prevented new hospital building and blocked large-scale technology purchases.

The CON federal mandate was repealed in 1987, however, and federal funding for CON efforts was eliminated under the Reagan Administration, which opposed the policy. Fourteen states almost immediately discontinued their CON programs entirely, but 34 states maintain some form of CON program to this day. Most of the CON programs still in place, however, have nowhere near their original breadth and scope. Existing laws concentrate primarily on the building of long-term care and outpatient facilities, especially those owned by physicians. Their main purpose is to monitor and prevent unnecessary and inappropriate care resulting from self-referral by physicians to facilities they own.

Other efforts to assess technologies, particularly at the federal level, have had similarly checkered histories. The congressional Office of Technology Assessment, created in 1972, was eliminated in 1995 after it had conducted hundreds of studies on health technology—many critical of the laissez-faire approach in the United States to paying for treatments not yet proven to be fully cost effective. To this day, Medicare rules limit the federal government from assessing new (or old) medical technologies for the purposes of preventing reimbursement if the use of the technology has become "standard practice." The Agency for Health Care Research and Policy (AHRQ) and the Patient Centered Outcomes Research Institute (PCORI)—the quasi-independent, nonprofit organization established under the Affordable Care Act—face similar restrictions on their ability to assess treatments, technologies and health services from the payment and reimbursement perspective. Although they can, and do, compare treatments and services, they cannot do so in a way that assesses cost-effectiveness.

Health Information Technology

In sharp contrast to the federal and state efforts to restrain technology under CON programs, the federal government initiated a large-scale effort to encourage adoption of health information technology and electronic health records (EHRs) out of a perceived need to modernize the use of clinical information within the health care system. Concerned that providers across the country had been slow to adopt health information technology to support clinical delivery of health care, Congress in 2009 enacted a multi-year plan to directly subsidize the purchase of EHR systems by hospitals and doctors through the Medicare and Medicaid programs, subject to a specific set of requirements that providers make "meaningful use" of the technology. The so-called HITECH (Health Information Technology for Economic and Clinical Health) Act was part of the federal stimulus package tied to the recession of 2007-2009, and was variously couched as a way to stimulate technology innovation and development, pave the way for the health care reform effort that eventually followed, and boost job growth. More than $37 billion in incentives to adopt electronic health record systems was ultimately paid out to health care providers from 2011 through 2017 to defray the costs of adoption, out of recognition that the benefits would ultimately flow to patients and consumers, and society as a whole.

Although EHR adoption is now widespread throughout U.S. health care, the initiative has yet to accomplish its goal of creating fully interoperable health information exchange, either among entities in the health care system, or between these entities and patients. Other promised benefits also remain elusive.[53] For example, clinicians continue to struggle with the perceived poor usability of EHR systems, and the redesign of work flow to accommodate them. Evidence on whether EHRs and other forms of health information technology improve care and save money, or add to costs, is mixed.

Durable Medical Equipment

The government's payment for durable medical equipment (DME) under Medicare provides a third relevant example of payment policy affecting technology adoption and use. DME refers to medical products that a doctor prescribes for a patient to use in his or her home, such as blood sugar monitors, infusion pumps, or sleep apnea devices. In Medicare, the Centers for Medicare and Medicaid Services (CMS) traditionally paid 80 percent of an allowed purchase price for a DME item, while the patient paid 20 percent. However, independent studies and government audits revealed that the system encouraged wildly inflated prices for DME that often exceeded prices in the private market. As a result, in 2003, Congress mandated that Medicare launch a competitive bidding program for some types of durable medical equipment, as well as for prosthetics, orthotics and certain supplies.

In this program, suppliers bid to provide certain medical equipment and supplies at fixed prices to Medicare enrollees in designated competitive bidding areas. Research undertaken by the Health Care Cost Institute (HCCI) has found that the Competitive Bidding Program lowered Medicare costs on durable medical equipment (DME), bringing spending down to levels experienced by many commercial payers.[54]

The Growing Role of Measures Linked to Payment

Quality measurement is integral to the shift from volume to value and payment based on value and outcomes. Increasingly, fee-for service payment bonuses to providers for making quality improvements, and penalties based on falling short of quality targets, are based on specific quality measures. For example, in some arrangements, primary care providers stand to gain bonuses when they score highly on measures that assess both the percentage of patients they screen for blood pressure and high blood sugar, and the percentage of patients with high blood pressure or diabetes who have those conditions under control. In health care systems that integrate both the provision of care and the financing of it, such as Kaiser Permanente, a substantial portion of a physician's payment may be contingent on performance on a set of quality metrics.

The quality measurement enterprise in the United States has been evolving over the past 20 years, and now has a complex infrastructure. Generally speaking, the use of technologies that could enhance a quality or performance score is implicit in many quality measures, but is not an explicit part of the vast majority of quality measures. Consider a prominent quality intervention and measure such as the penalty imposed by CMS on hospitals that have excessive rates of readmitting patients within 30 days. Such a measure does not explicitly "reward" hospitals for using remote monitoring of a patient's congestive heart failure to minimize the likelihood of readmission, but implicitly it does so.

Technologies for a Distributed Health Care System

At present, there is no overall public or private plan to subsidize or promote the purchase or adoption of technologies that would underpin a system of Health Care Without Walls. The absence of any such plan is probably appropriate, due to a lack of systematic health technology assessment, particularly in the digital health area. (Health technology assessment is "the systematic evaluation of properties, effects, and/or impacts of health technology. Its main purpose is to inform technology-related policy-making in health care, and thus improve the uptake of cost-effective new technologies and prevent the uptake of technologies that are of doubtful value for the health system."[55]

In fact, for many emerging technologies that would support a system of more distributed health care, there is not yet a substantial base of evidence on either effectiveness or cost effectiveness. Efforts such as that of NODEHealth (the Network of Digital Evidence in Health), a diverse group of academic innovation centers, industry, investors, and entrepreneurs, are under way to develop a robust evidence base for digital health, but as yet only a handful of these technologies have been evaluated. In part because of the lag in recognition of technology costs in the payment system as described above, it is also unclear what the return on investment would be for a provider or other payer—for example, to purchase a system pairing a wearable device and smart phone to track blood pressure and blood glucose levels for patients with diabetes and hypertension who are enrolled in a given health plan.

Moreover, and as discussed further below, some payers have been understandably reluctant to pay for such novel approaches and tools—or even for older telemedicine tools and infrastructure—out of fear that they will add to costs without improving health, or that they will fail to reduce medical expenditures while not harming health. As a result, a primary goal of the payment and reimbursement work stream has been to consider ways to incentivize the shift to a more flexible health care system that allows for more distributed care, and adoption of the technology that would enable it, while avoiding the addition of more cost and complexity to the payment system or further incentivizing delivery of low-value services.

The work stream thus considered two key questions: how best to pay for the acquisition of technology, and how best to pay for delivery of the services enabled by technology, to incentivize the move to more distributed care. The work stream also considered these questions against the backdrop of a U.S. health care system that is transitioning—albeit slowly—from fee-for-service payment to value-based payment. It sought to find ways to encourage that transition while also encouraging adoption of new technologies—in effect, nudging health care providers along a "glide path" to greater value-based payment and enhanced use of innovative technologies at the same time.

The work stream determined that the overall goals of the movement from volume-based payment to value-based payment in support of "health care without walls" approaches should be to create new payment models that achieve the following:

- Drive innovation in the movement of care to more distributed and convenient settings when appropriate for, and desired by, patients;

- Encourage attention to be paid to upstream drivers of health;

- Incentivize the efficient use of resources and reduce or restrain the growth of overall system costs;

- Sharply reduce inappropriate and unnecessary care, while also addressing under treatment of appropriate and necessary care;

- Improve the quality and safety of care;

- Compensate providers fairly, and where appropriate, shift more financial risk, and potential for upside rewards, to health systems and providers for meeting the objectives described above;

- Increase efforts at fraud prevention;

- Hold providers accountable for quality and outcomes, and in particular, the outcomes that are important for patients;

- Improve patients' health, rather than simply providing care;

- Innovate in putting more financial resources directly in the hands of patients to give them greater incentives to undertake self-care and improve their own health.

Payment efficiency

In the most radical vision of new payment models, CPT codes, complex formula-based fee schedules, and the accompanying layers of bureaucracy that accompany them would all disappear. They would be replaced by approaches such as global budgeting, "bundled" payments, and full per member/per month capitated payment. As noted, a transition to forms of payment more along these lines is under way, but is occurring slowly. The work group supports the acceleration of the transition, but understands that it must be deliberate and informed where possible by evidence—and that during the transition, fee-for service payment will continue to be the main mechanism by which many providers will be paid.

The Affordable Care Act established the CMS Center for Medicare and Medicaid Innovation, or CMMI, to test new payment models and delivery approaches along the lines described above, and private payers have also adopted a range of payment innovations. As a result, the Health Care Payment Learning and Action Network, a private-public collaborative, determined that 29 percent of total U.S. health care payments were tied to alternative payment models (APMs) in 2016, up from 23 percent in 2015. The APMs included shared savings, shared risk, bundled payment, and population-based payments. Notably, 43 percent of health care dollars in 2016 flowed via traditional fee-for-service or other legacy payment not linked to quality at all while 28 percent of dollars were primarily FFS-based but had some form of pay-for-performance or care-coordination incentives attached. The LAN estimated total APM-linked payments in 2016 at $354.5 billion nationally—much of it channeled through an estimated 600 ACOs.[56]

Alternative payment models have included a raft of approaches, such as bundled payments for such conditions as hip and knee replacements, in which payment is split among a range of clinicians and the hospital or other setting where surgery is performed.[57] For physicians and other clinicians, CMS is in the midst of implementing a new Quality Payment Program that, for now, largely preserves FFS payments, links such payments increasingly to quality, performance and resource use metrics, and encourages providers to move into Advanced Alternative Payment Models, or AAPMs.[58] Among these may be more physician-focused alternative payment models that are synergistic with distributed health care delivery, such as the "Hospital at Home-Plus" model devised by the Mount Sinai (New York) health system that was recommended for adoption by the Physician-Focused Payment Model Technical Advisory Committee (PTAC) created under MACRA (although ultimately not recommended for automatic adoption into the program by the Secretary, as described further below).[59]

Hospital at home programs have flourished in many other countries, but their use in the United States is still limited. This remains true despite strong evidence that well-monitored, at-home treatment can be safer, cheaper, and more effective than traditional hospital care. Superior outcomes are especially possible for patients who are vulnerable to hospital-acquired infections and other complications of inpatient care. Renewed interest has been sparked in recent years in the approach, largely based on the operational success of the program in various settings. The program was launched initially in 1994 at Johns Hopkins and has since been adapted by other hospitals and health systems, such as Mount Sinai (see regulatory chapter for a further discussion of the model). The model significantly incorporates telemedicine, remote monitoring and other distributed care modalities.[60]

The saga of Mount Sinai's version, known as Hospital at Home Plus, illustrates the multiple ways payment and regulatory obstacles militate against innovation. After a successful CMS demonstration of the Mount Sinai model, the approach was approved in 2017 as proposed by the Physician-Focused Payment Model Technical Advisory Committee, or PTAC. PTAC then referred the model on to the Secretary of Health and Human Services, for adoption into the Medicare program as a Physician-Focused Payment Model under the Quality Payment Program in Medicare. Such a designation would have permitted physicians, clinicians and others to effectively be paid more than they would through the traditional Medicare program, as they would be participating in a value-based alternative payment model under the MACRA law.

However, in June 2018, the Secretary of Health and Human Services, Alex Azar, wrote that HHS "will not implement this model as proposed." Instead, he wrote, the department was "exploring a model that allows beneficiaries with certain acute illnesses or exacerbated chronic diseases to receive hospital-level services in their homes." [61]

In the meantime, Mount Sinai has encountered other payment-related obstacles as well. Although it has been able to offer its Hospital at Home program in partnership with both commercial health plans and Medicare Advantage plans, it cannot in effect do so under the traditional Medicare program, since the traditional program provides no mechanism for billing for key aspects of the model, such as telehealth to patients "hospitalized" at home, visits to them by community paramedicine units, or even oxygen for acutely ill patients. The Mount Sinai hospital at home program has considered simply bearing the cost of these services and, in effect, "giving" them to patients, but hasn't done so for fear that such a "gift" might well amount to an illegal inducement under the federal Anti-Kickback statute.

Such Catch-22 situations are not unusual, given the complex structure of existing payment models that were tailored for a different era. Clearly, there is a need to rationalize Medicare and other payment systems to permit innovation that would foster more distributed care.

The Quest for New Payment Models

As a result, in considering the question of payment for technology in the move to more distributed health care, the payment Work Stream sought to understand how to incentivize both the uptake of technology and greater efficiency in health care delivery at the same time. Conversely, it sought to avoid encouraging the provision of additional services, rather than the substitution of one set of services for another. The work stream noted that much of the impetus to adopt new technologies is occurring now within capitated systems. Such systems inherently have strong incentives to displace inefficient forms of care delivery with more efficient ones. At Kaiser Permanente, for example, 52 percent of the more than 100 million patient encounters each year are now virtual visits.[62] Similarly, the Veterans Administration, a budgeted entity, has broadly adopted telemedicine, as discussed in detail in both the technology and regulatory chapters in this report.[63]

Nonetheless, the work stream agreed that since many payers and providers are not likely to adopt capitated or shared risk models in the near future, both the federal government and private payers will have to adopt incentives in fee-for-service payment that somehow encourage adoption of technology without prompting increases in utilization that do not lead to better health outcomes. Otherwise, the lack of ability to recover the costs incurred in the deployment of technology will continue to hobble its adoption. A valuable lesson in this regard is the experience of telemedicine and telehealth. Despite its initial use in health care as far back as the 1960s,[64] there has been comparatively slow adoption over time, and telehealth is only now coming into broad use in health care. The following section offers an extended case example of payment for telehealth to illustrate the types of problems that may need to be overcome to deploy these and other technologies more broadly into health care.

Telemedicine/Telehealth and Payment

Although the concepts and capabilities of telemedicine and telehealth date back approximately 50 years, adoption is only now advancing significantly as consumers and providers become more willing to use it and payers agree to pay for it, at least in limited ways. For example, according to the National Business Group on Health, 90 percent of large, primarily self-insured employers offer telemedicine to their employees, and another eight percent of employers plan to offer telemedicine in the next three years.[65] Still, federal, state and private sector payment policies for telehealth and telemedicine vary greatly and carry various restrictions.

A core obstacle for many payers is the fear that telehealth will be an add-on—and not a substitute service—that will trigger additional services at additional costs, with clear evidence of their clinical value. Some payers have also been deterred by lack of strong interest by consumers in receiving care via telehealth, although consumers' attitudes may be changing. Payers may also have perceived little need to invest in telemedicine by the fact that, until recently, relatively few provider systems have adopted telehealth and telemedicine outside of primary care. This reality, too, is changing, as systems like the University of Virginia, Intermountain, Dartmouth-Hitchcock, and others employ telehealth across multiple specialties.

Telehealth in Medicare

Until recently, Medicare payment policy could be described as erecting a huge wall against broad use of telehealth, except in limited circumstances. The existence of this wall has no doubt been a rate-limiting factor throughout the decades in the use of telehealth. However, chinks are now being carved in that wall, both via legislation and rulemaking, such that use of telehealth is likely to become increasingly more commonplace in the treatment of Medicare enrollees.

Medicare currently pays for telehealth "visits" under Part B, but with limits, and under the condition that the services substitute for an in-person encounter. (Notably, this limitation does not preclude follow-up in-person visits.) Under current law, the Medicare program generally restricts payment for telehealth services based on the type of service provided, the location of services, the type of institution, and the type of health care provider. [66,67]

More specifically, Medicare reimbursement in traditional fee-for-service Medicare can occur only when patients present at an "originating site"—defined as a health care setting (not a patient's home) that is (a) located in a designated rural health professional shortage area; (b) not in a metropolitan statistical area, or (c) a site participating in a federal telemedicine demonstration project. Urban hospitals and community health centers located in urban areas thus do not qualify as originating sites. As such, Medicare's restrictive payment policy limits the utility of telemedicine in urban health-care settings. Contrary to the growing use of telehealth within the VA system, Medicare's fee-for-service policies disallow telehealth visits directly into or from a patient's home.

At the same time, there are exceptions that allow broader use of telemedicine under certain circumstances and payment arrangements. Medicare Advantage (MA) plans, for example, have been permitted more flexibility to modify Medicare's payment rules for telemedicine. In new rules for 2019 and beyond, the government has expanded that flexibility as it applies to telemedicine but also other supplemental benefits that MA plans may wish to offer enrollees. These include chronic care management interventions and benefits that "have a reasonable expectation of improving or maintaining the health or overall function of the chronically ill enrollee and may not be limited to being primarily health related benefits." The new rules would also allow MA plans more flexibility to offer "non-medical" benefits such as meal delivery and transport to medical appointments. This new flexibility is an initial foray in the MA program government into allowing plans to address the "upstream" social determinants of health.

In the context of telemedicine, the new rule may move Medicare Advantage plans away from their practice to date of adhering to the originating site rule in fee-for-service Medicare—a practice that they have presumably maintained to ensure consistency and to restrain costs. The CMS rules also allow MA plans more flexibility in meeting network adequacy standards, a change that will in all likelihood permit plans to use advanced practice nurses, physician assistants and other non-physician providers more liberally, including in the delivery of telemedicine services.

CMS has also recently implemented a telehealth expansion "waiver" for Next Generation Accountable Care Organizations. The waiver eliminates the rural geographic component of originating site requirements, allows the originating site to include a beneficiary's home, and also allows for the use of "asynchronous" telehealth services (i.e., transfer of digital images and other data for interpretation at a remote site by health professionals) in the specialties of teledermatology and teleophthalmology. The waiver applies only to beneficiaries aligned with a Next Generation ACO and for services furnished by a Next Generation Participant or Preferred Provider who is approved to use the waiver.

Medicare's Chronic Care Management Program (also known as the Connected Care Initiative) is another exception to policies that have generally militated against the use of telehealth. This initiative[68]—which offers beneficiaries with chronic conditions access to special services, including 24/7 access to a health professional in emergency situations—places no restrictions on the use of telemedicine. It also allows for reimbursement of telemedicine visits regardless of originating site. Patients can be located anywhere and receive services from almost any provider or facility.

CMS also recently included provisions in two of its 2018 payment rules aimed at expanding telehealth services in the Medicare program. These include new physician fee schedule updates for remote monitoring and for telemedicine use related to lung-cancer screening, health risk assessments, psychotherapy in crisis situations, and chronic care management. In addition, the new rules allow physicians to use telehealth to meet clinical-practice improvement activities and receive incentive payments through the Quality Payment Program.

Meanwhile, Congress has contemplated—and in one recent instance, enacted—legislation to expand the use of telehealth in Medicare. In February 2018, it enacted as part of a federal budget agreement the "Creating High-Quality Results and Outcomes Necessary to Improve Chronic Care Act (the CHRONIC Care Act); the provision was signed into law by President Donald J. Trump on February 9, 2018. The law expands the use of telemedicine for treatment of stroke and dialysis patients in traditional Medicare, as well as for use within accountable care organizations and Medicare Advantage Plans. It also lifts the requirement that telehealth services for these patients apply only to patients in rural areas and small towns. Furthermore, the law removes geographic requirements as they relate to telemedicine use in Medicare Accountable Care Organizations (ACOs), and explicitly allows beneficiaries assigned to Medicare Shared Savings Programs or other Medicare ACOs to receive allowable telehealth services in their homes. Finally, it modifies the rules applying to Medicare Advantage plans, allowing them to include telehealth services in their annual bids.

Another proposed piece of legislation, the CONNECT for Health Act of 2017 (S. 1016) would go further than the CHRONIC Care Act to enact broader telehealth reforms. In addition to the provisions in CHRONIC, the CONNECT for Health Act would expand the use of telehealth in rural health clinics, community health center sites, and the Indian Health Service. The proposed legislation would also create a remote patient monitoring benefit for certain high-risk patients and allow use of telehealth and remote monitoring in bundled payments and for mental health. CONNECT would mandate evaluations of telehealth in CMS and in other delivery system reform demonstrations undertaken by CMS and the Center for Medicare and Medicaid Innovation (CMMI). However, the legislation's prospects in the current Congress are unknown.

Finally, with respect to remote monitoring—arguably one form of telehealth—in July 2018 CMS proposed a change to Medicare's home health payment system that will facilitate the adoption of remote monitoring in the provision of home health care. Currently, outlays for remote monitoring technology cannot be included in the cost reports that home health agencies file with CMS so that the agency can determine if home health care providers are being paid appropriately. Under CMS' proposed changes, which would take effect in 2020, CMS would allow the cost of remote patient monitoring to be reported by home health agencies as allowable costs on the Medicare cost report form. Although home health providers would not be directly reimbursed for the installation and use of equipment, the change would in effect enable home health providers' outlays related to remote monitoring to be captured in the payment system. In a news release, CMS said the change would "help foster the adoption of emerging technologies by home health agencies and result in more effective care planning, as data is shared among patients, their caregivers, and their providers." [69]

Telehealth in Medicaid

It's no exaggeration to say that reimbursement policies for telehealth provided under Medicaid are a patchwork quilt that vary widely from one state to another.

States have broad flexibility under federal rules to incorporate telemedicine services into their Medicaid programs, and all but one (New Hampshire) has avoided duplicating Medicare "originating site" rule in either fee-for-service Medicaid or Medicaid managed care plans. That said, many states continue to impose limits on the type of facility from which provider-to-patient telehealth emanates and where it is received. In some states, for example, telehealth that is received in, or emanates from, a patient's home is restricted. Such restrictions impose a de facto limit on the use of remote monitoring in patients' homes as well as conventional video consultations between home-bound patients and providers.

The Center for Connected Health Policy has issued a report each year for the past five years on "State Telehealth Laws and Reimbursement Policies."[70] Its April 2018 report finds, overall, that although states continue to expand telehealth reimbursement under Medicaid, most have retained restrictions and limitations. Notably, any type of medical consultation, care, or advice provided by email, telephone, and fax, are rarely considered telehealth within statutory and regulatory definitions. States either are silent on these forms of medical information exchange, or explicitly exclude coverage of them. What's more, Medicaid reimbursement for live video telehealth visits continues to exceed reimbursement for remote patient monitoring and "store-and-forward" technologies (the electronic transmission of medical information, such as digital images, documents, and pre-recorded videos through secure email transmission, typically among medical professionals), although reimbursement of store-and-forward technologies and remote monitoring is slowly increasing.

As of 2018, 49 states and the District of Columbia provide reimbursement for some form of live video in Medicaid fee-for-service, but what they reimburse for, and how, varies. New Jersey Medicaid, for example, only reimburses for tele-psychiatry, while California reimburses for live video across almost all specialties. Fifteen states reimburse for store-and-forward forms of telehealth; 20 states reimburse for remote patient monitoring (another four states have laws requiring that Medicaid fee-for-service pay for remote monitoring or establish a pilot program to do so, but no official state policy putting these requirements into effect). Nine Medicaid programs (Alaska, Arizona, Hawaii, Illinois, Minnesota, Mississippi, Missouri, Virginia and Washington) reimburse for all three modes of telehealth: live video, store-and-forward and remote patient monitoring. Teledentistry coverage in Medicaid grew significantly in 2017, with seven states adding it.

In addition to their different policies on live video reimbursement, many states have restrictions on the following:

- The type of services that can be reimbursed (such as "visits" that originate in a clinician's office, or in an inpatient setting).

- The type of provider whose services can be reimbursed (such as a physician, nurse, or physician assistant).

- The location of the patient, whether in an inpatient setting, a medical office, or home or other community setting.

Reimbursement limitations imposed by state Medicaid programs on store-and-forward technologies and exchanges are highly variable. For example, California only reimburses for store-and-forward exchanges conducted in tele-dermatology, tele-ophthalmology and teledentistry. And several state Medicaid plans only reimburse for tele-radiology (which is commonly reimbursed, and not always considered telehealth).

For the states allowing payment for remote patient monitoring, the most common restrictions are as follows:

- Only offering reimbursement to home health agencies, rather than other types of providers;

- Restricting the clinical condition for which symptoms can be monitored;
- Limiting the type of monitoring device and information that can be collected.

For example, Colorado only permits patients to receive services for congestive heart failure, chronic obstructive pulmonary disease, asthma, or diabetes. In Minnesota, payment is restricted to skilled nursing visits and in that state's "Elderly Waiver and Alternative Care" programs.

In addition to provision for reimbursement of the actual delivery of telehealth services, most states (31) allow reimbursement for "originating site" facility and transmission fees associated with telehealth—to cover incidental "hosting" expenses.

Telehealth and Private Payers

Almost all major insurers and health plans now reimburse for telehealth, but with restrictions, and their policies differ widely. Several dozen CPT codes and code modifiers cover specific telehealth uses and services, but doctors can also bill under other patient-visit CPT codes for telehealth visits.

Many private payers have been particularly wary of telemedicine, as evidence suggests that direct-to-consumer telehealth services can prompt new use of medical services, and thus drive up spending.[71] Payers informally describe a telehealth visit as resulting in a "punt." For example, in a telehealth visit, a provider may recommend that a patient later consult with his or her primary care physician, or go to a hospital emergency department. The payment for the telehealth visit then results in an add-on to the visits that occur, often directly as a result, elsewhere in the health care system.

RAND Corp. researchers identified this same phenomenon in a study released in 2017.[72] The study analyzed the behavior of more than 300,000 people with generous medical benefits (including telemedicine) from the California Public Employee Retirement System (CalPERS). It found that just 12 percent of the telemedicine visits *replaced* visits to doctor's offices or emergency rooms, while 88 percent represented new use of medical services.bbThe research focused primarily on care for acute respiratory conditions, including sinus infections and bronchitis -- among the most common reasons people seek care from telehealth providers. For each episode of acute respiratory infection, the cost of telehealth services were about 50 percent lower than a physician office visit, and less than 5 percent the cost of a visit to an emergency department. However, overall savings from substitution of one service for another in this population was outweighed by the additional costs of new use of telehealth services, which averaged $45 per telehealth user.

Although the focus on the selected conditions described above means that the study is not necessarily representative of all potential uses of telemedicine, it nonetheless raised concerns about broad reimbursement of telemedicine for comparatively minor illnesses in the absence of other incentives to control utilization. The study suggested that, in such situations, the greater convenience of "around-the-clock" access to physicians via telephone or videoconferencing would add to costs. Earlier, the same RAND researchers reported similar findings on the use of retail clinics—another avenue of convenient consumer access to health care—in a study published in 2016.[73] They estimated that 58 percent of visits to retail clinics for low-severity illnesses constituted new uses of medical services, rather than substitutes for visiting a doctor's office or emergency department, and thus also added to overall costs.

Notwithstanding payers' concerns about the potential cost-increasing potential of telehealth, lawmakers in many states are pushing private payers to cover more telehealth services. During the 2017 legislative session, lawmakers in 44 states debated some 200 telehealth-related pieces of legislation. Most of the proposed bills addressed reimbursement, pertaining to both Medicaid and private payers, although others—such as one adopted in Texas—removed the "physical visit" requirement that barred physicians from conducting telemedicine visits with patients whom they had not yet seen in-person first. Currently, 35 jurisdictions have laws in place that govern private-payer telehealth reimbursement policies. And, according to the American Telemedicine Association (ATA), as of June 2018 40 state legislatures had either enacted or debated proposed legislation allowing for full or partial telemedicine parity.[74] These parity provisions typically require that coverage and reimbursement for a telehealth-delivered service be equal to care delivered in-person.

Many state lawmakers have also proposed legislation that would direct licensure boards to establish standards for telehealth. A few states have also begun introducing legislation or proposing regulation that would allow for telehealth to be counted towards network adequacy requirements for both Medicaid managed care plans and the private sector.

Lessons Learned in Telehealth Regulation

The complex picture described above—of a veritable patchwork quilt of provisions for coverage of telehealth among payers and across the 50 states—constitutes an object lesson in the evolution of Health Care Without Walls. It is difficult to imagine the nation making much progress in the adoption of more distributed care if all new types of technology-based interventions are subject to a similarly uneven—and in many respects, illogical—pattern of coverage. Although it is clear that foot-dragging on coverage of telehealth has prevented a surge of telehealth utilization, the question is at what cost to health and health care? It is beyond the scope of this paper to answer that question, but important to pose it, in part to make the case for approaching future technologies and questions about coverage and payment in a very different way.

The Case and Cause of Rural Health Improvement

One priority objective for the Health Care Without Walls initiative is to improve access, quality-of-care, and affordability in rural areas and other medically underserved parts of the country. A report by the Bipartisan Policy Center, released in January 2018[75]—and based in part on in-depth conversations with rural health leaders—argues that a shift from traditional institutions and modes of care to alternative platforms, delivery systems, and payment models is the best way to improve care in rural America. Such reconfigured systems would in all likelihood take advantage of technologies such as telehealth as well as in-home care to deliver care in cost-effective ways.

Stakeholders interviewed by the Bipartisan Policy Center identified these current payment- and reimbursement-related factors as the main obstacles to advancing telehealth in rural areas:

- The lack of parity between telemedicine and in-person visit reimbursements;

- The lack of common standards among payers for what types of telehealth qualify for reimbursement;

- Rapidly changing/evolving policies and practices by private payers on reimbursement;

- Limits by both private and public payers on what types of telemedicine services they will reimburse;

- Licensure laws that limit telemedicine's reach, since state licensure rules can prevent providers from practicing virtually across state lines (see the Health Care Without Walls Regulatory Work Stream chapter for a discussion of this issue); and

- Poor or non-existent broadband infrastructure. Expanded and less expensive broadband internet would enhance telemedicine and make it less expensive to provide (again, see the regulatory chapter for a longer discussion).

Assuming that many of these issues were dealt with—for example, licensure—technologies such as telehealth and telemedicine could be more broadly implemented, and linked to payment and legislative reforms to reconfigure rural health care delivery for the 21st century.

Consider the case of Critical Access Hospitals (CAHs), one of four types of Medicare classifications for hospitals that serve rural communities (the others are sole provider hospitals, Medicare-dependent hospitals, and rural referral centers). Although not all rural hospitals are under severe financial pressure, many are – and as a group, critical access hospitals, which have the oldest plant and equipment, have been among the hardest hit.[76] However, as a detailed 2010 study of these hospitals noted, "Many rural hospitals are the only hospital facility in their community and their survival is vital to ensure timely access to health care." [77]As a result, both the federal government and states for several years have been assessing how best to ensure access to care in rural areas, through CAHs and the other types of rural health care providers.

The nation's 1,340 critical access hospitals operate under a Medicare designation dating back to 1997, which permits special payment arrangements for hospitals with no more than 25 inpatient beds, and that are at least 15 miles by secondary road and 35 miles by primary road from another hospital. Under current Medicare rules, CAHs are not paid under Medicare's prospective payment systems for inpatient or outpatient care, but rather are paid under a "cost-plus" structure that reimburses them at 101 percent of reasonable costs. In addition, payments to a CAH for inpatient services are not subject to ceilings on hospital inpatient operating costs, or the 1-day or 3-day preadmission payment window provisions applicable to hospitals paid under Medicare's prospective payment systems.

A 2013 Inspector General's report[78] observed that nearly two-thirds of CAHs would not meet the locations requirements described above if they were required to re-enroll. Without the extra payment under Medicare, many would undoubtedly fail. Given relatively low patient censuses and the financial stresses suffered by many of these hospitals, it is not clear that all of them are needed in rural communities. However, states are concerned about a repeat of what happened in the 1980s and 1990s, when hundreds of small rural hospitals closed due to market forces and payment policies, creating gaps in the health care services in rural areas.

A number of plans have been introduced in Congress and elsewhere to transform CAHs into new care delivery model facilities. Thus, the potential exists to employ telehealth and other virtual and distributed care approaches as part of this transformation. The proposed Save Rural Hospitals Act, for example, would allow CAHs to transform into outpatient-care hospitals and to provide urgent outpatient care.

Similarly, the proposed Rural Emergency Acute Care Hospital Act would allow CAHs in some communities to become rural emergency centers. Under draft legislation proposed by the National Rural Health Association, CAHs would be required to join an accountable care organization (ACO) within three to five years. And in 2017, CMS approved a Pennsylvania demonstration project that will supply $25 million over four years to support the implementation of an all-payer global budget for the state's rural hospitals, permitting them to innovate in a number of ways. A similar approach was recently adopted in Maryland under that state's all-payer rate-setting system. (Further discussion of these two models is in the recommendations section below).

The Bipartisan Policy Center report underscores the view that a shift away from fee-for-service payment toward value-based payment models provides rural providers the best opportunity to transform local delivery systems and improve access to care. The report also makes clear that Health Care Without Walls approaches – including health care work force changes that makes greater use of advanced practice nurses, physician assistants, and community health workers—will be important avenues for connecting rural health organizations to larger health systems, improving both their financial viability and ability to serve rural health needs.

The Health Care Without Walls payment and reimbursement Work Stream expressed the view that rural areas of the United States constitute a vitally important test bed for these and other distributed care approaches. New models of care could reduce the existing inpatient hospital footprint of rural hospitals; add observation beds and emergency transportation systems; add telehealth capabilities that would link rural clinics and observation centers with larger health systems in urban areas; and pump resources into community-based health prevention and promotion activities.

As a result, the work stream formulated recommendations to advance distributed care in rural areas by building these capabilities into some existing payment and delivery transformation models, as set forth below.

Payment for the Future: Pursuing a "Glide Path" to New Payment Models

In its deliberations about what payment models might look like in the future, the work stream considered both idealized and pragmatic approaches to models that would best support the move to more distributed care. In an idealized world, if the U.S. health care system were globally budgeted, or composed largely or almost exclusively of capitated systems, the system or systems would inherently have incentives to take up technologies that enabled them to provide care in more cost-effective ways—for example, by substituting a telehealth visit for a physical, in-person visit in appropriate instances.

However, the work stream concluded that it would be entirely impractical to wait for the day when most of the U.S. health care system has abandoned fee-for-service payment and shifted to global budgets in order to put these technologies in place. Hence, the work stream developed the notion of a "glide path"—creating payment incentives that would simultaneously encourage technology adoption, the move of health care to more distributed settings, and the ongoing transition to value-based payment.

Substantial effort has already been devoted to devising new value-based payment models that address these considerations, often for episodes of care that make use of specific technologies. For example, several submissions to the Physician-Focused Payment Model Technical Advisory Committee (PTAC) for proposed new physician focused payment models under MACRA have taken this tack. One example is Project Sonar, a care management program developed by community-based physicians to improve the management of patients with chronic inflammatory bowel disease.[79] Part of the program is a web and mobile-based platform that exchanges text messages to patients, and captures patient response data that is fed directly into electronic health records. Although the model was recommended to the Secretary of

Health and Human Services for limited testing for Medicare payment to physicians by PTAC, then-Secretary Tom Price declined to endorse the model,[80] apparently out of a misunderstanding that it would necessarily involve a specific proprietary technology rather than a general technology-based approach.

The Health Care Without Walls payment Work Stream sought to frame proposals for new payment models that would incentivize use of technologies in general to make care more efficient, effective, cost-effective, and convenient, without necessarily paying directly for those technologies. It also sought a way to incentivize patients to use these technologies to take a greater role in their own care, particularly through self-care, and especially for the purposes of primary and secondary prevention of disease. And as stated above, these new payment approaches should be structured to provide a "glide path" toward value-based care models that link payment to the outcomes of greatest interest to patients.

The work stream considered, but rejected as less desirable, approaches that would specifically be directed at technology investments, such as tax write-offs for health systems investing in certain types of technology expenditures, or "meaningful use"—style incentives such as those designed to spur adoption of electronic health records under the federal HITECH law. Instead, it devised possible approaches in three categories, consisting of a series of incentives aimed at providers; at payers, including health plans and self-insured employers; and at patients and consumers.

Payment Incentives to Providers

For health care providers and systems, the work stream posited that a variety of new incentives could be created or expanded, as detailed below.

1) **Creation of "Technology-Enabled Episodes" (TEE's).** Current Procedural Terminology and Healthcare Common Procedure Coding System codes have not evolved to adequately track and pay for person-focused, technology-enabled care management. An alternative approach, combining features of episode-based payment or bundles with technology, would enable a range of providers to devise care and payment episodes making use of a range of information and other technologies in the delivery and management of care. Episodes could involve payment to physicians, as in the Project Sonar proposal described above, or to suppliers, such as care and benefit management companies. These episode-based payments could be made by both public payers such as Medicare and Medicaid, and private payers, including both commercial health plans and self-insured employers.

For example, CMS recently created coding and a fee schedule to compensate community organizations and others that furnish the Diabetes Prevention Program to Medicare enrollees—a Centers for Disease Control and Prevention-approved curriculum of training in long-term dietary change, increased physical activity and behavior change for weight control that has been proven to halt progression from pre-diabetes to diabetes.[81] Similarly, analogous approaches could be devised around care episodes in which mobile and other technologies play a central role. These episodes should be linked to care outcomes valued by patients (see measures section below).

2) **Creation and experimentation with other new payment models by the Center for Medicare and Medicaid Innovation (CMMI).** Congress could direct CMS and CMMI to expand the volume of demonstrations that included new technology enabled care management and delivery models, to determine whether these models can reduce Medicare expenditures while preserving or enhancing the quality of care. Priorities could include a "hospital at home" or similar model such as those proposed to PTAC by Mount Sinai health system in New York and Personalized Recovery Care,[82] a joint venture between the Marshfield Clinic and Contessa Health to the Physician-Focused Payment Model Technical Advisory Committee. The work stream applauds the fact that the Secretary intends for CMMI to spur innovation in models based on similar approaches, and that hospitals and health systems continue to expand and refine their hospital-at-home programs.

3) Creation of large-scale transformation grants to rural and safety net providers, such as critical access hospitals, to enable them to shift away from their current acute care models and toward becoming community-based health care providers that serve as telehealth facilitators, primary care clinics, substitute observation units for inpatient beds, and provide transport to larger hospitals in more urban settings as needed. The grants would be funded by taxpayers, but could be financed through payment offsets or assumptions about shifts in payment. For example, if a large enough sample of critical access hospitals were encouraged to transform to new care models over time, the Congressional Budget Office might estimate that declines in cost-plus reimbursement under Medicare for these hospitals would offset the amount of transformation grants and other subsidies to assist hospitals and communities in making the transition.

4) With respect to Medicare, the expansion of Medicare's "new technology add-on payments (NTAPs)" should be considered to cover additional technologies. As discussed above, these payments were created under the Medicare inpatient prospective payment hospital system to recognize the costs of new medical services and technologies until the Centers for Medicare and Medicaid Services (CMS) is able to incorporate the actual costs into updated prospective payment rates. An imperative will be to more closely define what constitutes "new" technology. Under the existing NTAP provision, "new" is generally defined by CMS as within two to three years following Food and Drug Administration (FDA) approval or market introduction, and the use of the new technology also must constitute a substantial clinical improvement over existing services. Given that many existing technologies that are not necessarily "new" are being adapted anew for use in health care, these definitions may need to be revisited.

5) Also with respect to Medicare, the "Advancing Care Information" performance measure set that is part of Medicare's Quality Payment Program for clinicians (and specifically, part of the Medicare Merit-Based Incentive Payment System (MIPS)), could be expanded to incentivize adoption of distributed care technologies.

6) In Medicare Part B, CMS could expand the list of providers eligible to receive Part B payment to recognize the opportunity for a range of caregivers to provide value in distributed care delivery models—for example, pharmacists.

7) The U.S. Department of Health and Human Services Office of the Inspector General (OIG) and the Centers for Medicare and Medicaid Services (CMS) could expand the Stark Law fraud and abuse safe harbor that permits physicians to accept donations of electronic health records from health systems, and apply it to donations of equipment to conduct telehealth, remote monitoring, and other technologies supporting more distributed care.

Other changes that could be undertaken by payers: Medicare and Medicaid, commercial health plans, and self-insured employers

The payment work stream conceptualized a number of changes in payment policy that could be undertaken by this disparate group of payers, and that would support the shift to more distributed care.

1) For example, new methodologies could be created to encourage payers to more quickly recognize the increased costs of certain technologies in fee-for-service reimbursement. Alternatively, commercial payers could emulate Medicare's new technology add-on payments. Payers could receive tax incentives for more quickly recognizing the costs of these technologies in payments to providers. A downside of these approaches is that they would link payment so closely to technologies, as distinct to the outcomes of greatest interest to patients that may or may not be enhanced by the use of technology.

2) To encourage the use of mobile and other technologies, CMS could change the Medicare Marketing Guidelines that apply to Medicare Advantage (MA, MA-PD), Medicare Prescription Drug Plans, and so-called Section 1876 cost plans, to permit such plans to give low-cost technologies as telehealth monitors to enrollees to allow for more distributed care.

3) Commercial payers could be allowed to count their own investments in new technologies enabling more provision of distributed care as a medical expense for the purposes of the Medical Loss Ratio, rather than as administrative or overhead costs.

4) Congress could change the tax laws so that employers could count contributions for technologies that patients could use in their homes— e.g., for telehealth consultations—as part of an employer-provided wellness programs (specifically, as defined under Section 213) and therefore given tax-free to eligible employees. To be excludable from income, the benefit must qualify as medical care as defined under Sec. 213.

5) If the so-called "Cadillac" tax enacted as part of the Affordable Care Act is ever enforced (it is now delayed until 2022), Congress could exempt investments and expenditures for tools and services to provide more distributed care from the tax.

Patients, Consumers, and Family Caregivers

An intriguing line of thought in the work stream was how to incentivize consumers, patients, and family caregivers to take up the use of technologies that could be clearly linked to improved outcomes, in part through greater self-care and behavior change.

As work stream leaders sketched the concept, they pointed to the fact that the current payment system primarily pays health care providers to "do" things to patients with the aim of making them better. However, particularly in the realm of chronic disease, much of what will either prevent illness, constitute effective secondary prevention, or result in better management of the condition rests in the hands of patients or consumers.

For example, pre-diabetes may be prevented from progressing to diabetes if individuals lose a modest amount of weight and eat healthier diets, and now (as discussed above) a new payment model supports payment to providers who will educate patients along these lines. What if a portion of dollars now directed at paying providers instead flowed to individuals and patients, to incentivize them to take steps to change, particularly if certain technologies, such as mobile apps, could help them achieve the necessary changes?

Consider the proliferation of tablets, health care apps, and related patient-facing technologies that constitute important aspects of the movement to more distributed care. In England, four of the trusts, or hospitals, within the National Health Service in 2017 began testing medical apps that help people monitor their health at home for such conditions as gestational diabetes,[83] reducing their need to visit a doctor. The apps are set to be rolled out to as many as four UK National Health Service trusts over the next year. For its part, the Veterans Health Administration has an online "app store" that provides VA-developed apps for patients—among them, "Annie," which sends text messages prompting veterans to track their health and reply back to let VA providers know how they are doing.

A question that some U.S. payers are now contemplating is whether or not it would be cost-effective to incentivize patients to use these apps and other technologies as a form of self-care, perhaps in tandem with their health insurance coverage, or in conjunction with their participation in a corporate wellness program. For example, a patient who regularly entered his or her blood glucose levels on an app could receive a small bonus payment—perhaps even via a mobile payment mechanism such as Venmo—once a week's worth of that activity were completed. A patient who maintained hemoglobin a1c at or near a targeted level for a month at a time would get a small additional reward. In this way, patients could be incentivized to undertake self-care as a form of secondary prevention. Another possibility is that payers could investigate using these types of incentives to enlist patients in primary prevention—e.g., incentivizing young and healthy patients to use fitness trackers or nutrition-oriented apps to maintain good eating and exercise habits and maintain healthy weights.

Other measures undertaken by payers that could stimulate the move toward more distributed care could include the following:

- Insurers could create value-based benefit design models that reduce consumer cost sharing in instances when more cost-efficient distributed care is used appropriately—for example, in substituting a telehealth visit or a visit to an urgent care center or emergency department.

- Medicare Advantage plans could offer enrollees supplemental benefits to encourage use of cost-effective distributed care, and waive cost-sharing or a small portion of the monthly premium.

- Commercial insurers, Medicare Advantage plans, Special Needs plans and Medicaid managed care organizations could provide remote monitoring, telehealth and other related technologies to enrollees at no out-of-pocket cost to themselves—or, as described above, could actually be encouraged to use these technologies as part of self-care through small payments or other incentives.

Building Out Payment Models and Accumulating an Evidence Base

It is beyond the scope of this work to fully flesh out the above proposals, to cost them out, or to analyze their political or other viability. However, many of these possible measures, along with the work stream recommendations presented below, could help stimulate ongoing delivery system and payment reforms that could arguably gain momentum over time.

For example, as private payers and Medicare's new Quality Payment Program encourage greater provider risk sharing, more opportunities will arise to initiate and test virtual and e-visits, telehealth consults, remote monitoring, wearable technologies, technology-assisted home care, real-time smart-phone tracking of health status, and ultimately the application of artificial intelligence, machine learning, and data analytics—all under the umbrella of risk contracts that prioritize coordinated care, better outcomes, and cost constraint. By the same token, these emerging technologies are likely to be employed under capitated risk contracts, bundled payments, and other alternative payment models.

NEHI's work stream participants believe that among the most potent strategies for accelerating the shift to a value-based system over the next decade *is* to enhance payment incentives for care that is delivered outside the walls of hospitals, doctor's offices, nursing homes, and rehab centers—and that uses the rapidly evolving technological tools that make such care possible. As discussed above, such incentives can and should be extended to both patients or consumers as well as providers. However, the participants also strongly believe that more distributed care approaches and technologies should be rigorously assessed for evidence that they improve care in cost-effective ways; that the benefits exceed the costs; and/or that they reduce costs without impairing high quality care. They also believe that returns on investments in technology should be assessed in a disciplined and systematic way, as detailed further below.

Payment and Reimbursement Recommendations

1) The transition to a more innovative and adaptive system of care in the U.S. that would support more distributed care and foster improved access while constraining costs, would best be achieved via global budgets, capitated systems of payment, and at-risk contracting. However, given the long transition under way from fee-for-service payment to alternative payment models, a "glide path" approach will be needed to incentivize the adoption and implementation of technology alongside steps toward greater risk-sharing among providers.

   As discussed in this chapter, such incentives could include payment incentives that reward care delivered through virtual visits and technology giveaways (such as iPads with pre-loaded chronic care management programs). However, these incentives should be structured to transition providers into value-based models designed to encourage the most appropriate types of care in the most appropriate settings, rather than a greater volume of care.

2) Alternative payment models such as these should be developed, implemented, tested, and studied. As the **CHRONIC Act described above is implemented**, the effects of enhancing telemedicine delivery in certain

aspects of care delivered to Medicare enrollees should be studied and evaluated. The federal government's Center for Medicare and Medicaid Innovation (CMMI) should launch additional pilot tests of distributed care, and permit its liberal use in the latest models of accountable care organizations (ACOs) that are based on substantial risk- and gain-sharing with providers.

3) As much as possible, sets of measures should be developed that tie payment to outcomes that matter to patients, including patient-reported outcomes—and particularly so for payment models designed to stimulate the move of care to more distributed settings. The National Quality Forum and other entities that develop, implement or vet quality and performance measures should consider whether the uptake and use of certain tools and technologies that enhance distributed care need to be more explicitly promoted by quality metrics. For example, tools that support hospital-at-home programs are a critical component of successful at-home care. Likewise, the recent approval by FDA of a device that greatly enhances the diagnosis of diabetic retinopathy in primary care is an example of a specific tool that could warrant incorporation in a diabetes care quality measure.

4) More attention should be focused throughout the health care system, and among payers, providers, and patients alike, on the social determinants of health—the primary upstream drivers of health status. Experiments that test inclusion of at-home social and behavior support—and mental health care if needed—as part of alternative payment model risk contracts should be prioritized.

5) The Accountable Health Communities cooperative agreements launched by CMMI, which currently number 32 sites, should be expanded to encompass distributed care. The initiative aims to bridge the gap between clinical care and community services by testing whether systematically identifying and addressing the health-related social needs (food insecurity and inadequate or unstable housing, for example) of Medicare and Medicaid beneficiaries, through screening, referral, and community navigation services, will impact health care costs and reduce utilization. Physician practices, behavioral health providers, clinics, and hospitals are charged with conducting health-related social needs screenings and making referrals to community services. Federal funds support the infrastructure and staffing needs of bridge

organizations, but don't currently pay for social services or innovative care models.

6) Public and private payers should develop and test payment models that provide actual financial incentives to individuals to engage in primary and secondary prevention and self-care, potentially enabled by technologies such as mobile health. Payers, insurers, and integrated systems also should experiment with providing people with **free tools and technologies to enhance their health and manage chronic illnesses**. Examples are wearables, iPads, and devices such as Amazon's Echo (Alexa) or Google Home as well as specific equipment to enhance monitoring at home. Such experiments should be closely monitored to gauge impact and outcomes.

7) **Value-based insurance design** should be tested, in both commercial insurance and Medicare Advantage plans, as a way to incentivize consumers to choose lower costs providers and modes of care (including telehealth and urgent care clinics) for routine care, in lieu of hospital-based or stand-alone emergency rooms or a doctor's office visit. For example, such care could be exempt from deductibles and require smaller co-pays. Some preventive care and community-based social support services could also be exempt from deductibles and co-pays.

8) To support the expansion and appropriate use of nonphysician providers and team-based care, quality and performance measurement should be adapted to permit all the persons in a team (physician and non-physician clinician) to be evaluated and scored together under the umbrella of an alternative payment model. Such an approach would reduce the burden of measurement and promote team-based and coordinated care.

9) To encourage the spread of **Hospital-at-Home programs**, the Secretary of Health and Human Services should test and ultimately approve a hospital at home model either as a Physician-Focused Payment Model under the Medicare Quality Payment Program, or as some other form of advanced alternative payment model. The Secretary of Health and Human Services has signaled its "keen interest" in such a model, provided that concerns about ensuring patient safety and avoiding potential misalignment of incentives (e.g., the absence of any financial penalty if a patient is "readmitted" to an actual hospital 30 days after a "hospital at home" episode) can be addressed. With the support of commercial payers and self-

insured employers, hospitals and health systems in the interim should make an aggressive push to expand hospital-at-home programs.

10) The Health Resources and Services Administration should recommend to Congress, and Congress should enact, **federal legislation that permits community health centers to more broadly experiment** with distributed care. CHCs are the primary care provider to 27 million mostly low-income Americans. Since they are primarily funded by and overseen by federal and state government, they offer an opportunity to be used to study new systems and modes of care. Congress in February 2018 renewed federal grant funding for CHCs for 2 years, and CHCs enjoy broad bipartisan support, making them a very appropriate test bed for distributed health care approaches.

11) CMS should evaluate the prospect of incorporating distributed care into ongoing dual eligible experiments and payment and delivery reforms. The **dual eligible population, which receives both** Medicare and Medicaid, is sicker and poorer than the average Medicare-only population. Serving dual eligibles, many of whom are low-income seniors and others of whom are younger people with disabilities, presents another opportunity for testing distributed modes of care, such as remote patient monitoring and telehealth visits. CMS should expand its special needs program (SNPs) for Medicare beneficiaries to encompass targeted care for the dual eligible population.

12) CMS should incentivize Medicare Advantage plans to test new models of care and payment, and to accelerate the transition to global budgets and at-risk contracting for providers. CMS also should expand the existing Medicare Value-Based Insurance Design model[84] to permit MA plans more leeway to test approaches to distributed forms of care coupled with lower cost-sharing for beneficiaries. As discussed above, CMS in 2018 issued new rules that will permit MA plans more flexibility in offering telehealth and non-medical benefits, many of which will almost certainly promote at-home care. The MA program presents even more opportunity, however, for experimentation that tests care outside the usual parameters and platforms of care.

13) **More states could seek a waiver from CMS to emulate Maryland's** all-payer rate setting system for hospital services, authorized by a federal waiver, which could provide a means of testing distributed health care approaches. Under the model, which builds on a longstanding CMS waiver that was

renewed under new terms in 2015, Maryland hospitals committed to achieving significant quality improvements, reducing hospitals' 30-day hospital readmissions rate and hospital acquired conditions (HAC) rate, and limiting all-payer per capita hospital growth, including inpatient and outpatient care, to 3.58 percent annually. The states' hospitals also agreed to limit annual Medicare per capita hospital cost growth to a rate lower than the national annual per capita growth rate per year for 2015-2018. Medicare is estimated to save at least $330 million from the model over the next five years. Notably, however, the jury is still out on whether Maryland's hospitals reduced utilization, as also was hoped.85 Meanwhile, the Care Redesign Program, a voluntary program within the Maryland All-Payer Model, advances efforts to redesign and better coordinate care in Maryland. The Care Redesign Program and the de facto global budget around hospital services in the state could also provide the incentive to test more distributed services, such as "Hospital at Home." Other states should consider emulating Maryland's model to test similar approaches.

14) Many states also have waivers to test care delivery and payment innovations under their Medicaid programs. More states should use "Section 1115" waivers, including Delivery System Reform Incentive Payment (DSRIP) waivers, to test ways to reduce hospital, nursing home and other forms of institutional care.

15) Congress should establish a grant program, possibly through CMMI, that assists **small rural hospitals** (especially critical access hospitals) in transitioning to new delivery models, testing them in conjunction with alternative payment models, and adopting telehealth and other "Health Care without Walls" approaches.

16) More states should partner with CMMI to replicate their own versions of the Pennsylvania Rural Health Model, under which that state seeks to increase rural Pennsylvanians' access to high-quality care and improve their health, while also reducing the growth of hospital expenditures across payers, including Medicare. The model anticipates saving Medicare an estimated $35 million over 7 years and limiting overall spending growth on inpatient and outpatient hospital services to 3.38 percent annually, while increasing the financial viability of rural Pennsylvania hospitals at the same time. The participating rural hospitals are paid based on all-payer global budgets from Medicare and participating private payers for inpatient and outpatient hospital-based services. In the meantime, the hospitals are redesigning

care delivery to improve quality of care and meet the health needs of their local communities, with the state's Department of Health as a key partner. CMS is to provide $25 million over four years to help Pennsylvania begin its implementation of the Model. The Pennsylvania model anticipates being an important test bed for telehealth and other distributed health care approaches.

17) More states could also partner with CMS and other payers along the lines of **Vermont's** All-Payer Accountable Care Organization (ACO) Model. In this case, the most significant payers—Medicare, Medicaid, and commercial health care payers—are part of a five-year experiment, which has the potential to be an important test bed for distributed care. Under the model, the majority of the state's providers are to operate under the same payment scheme. Coupled with a separate Medicaid waiver and other provisions of state law, including constraints on the growth of overall state health spending, the state has incentives to test whether distributed care approaches can substitute for more costly services and improve community-level care. If the results look promising by year three (2020), CMS should expand this model to other states wishing to test the same or similar approaches.

18) The federal government should actively encourage the use and assessment of telehealth and other technology enabled tools in **Programs of All-Inclusive Care for the Elderly, or PACE**, which is a unique capitated managed care benefit for the frail elderly. The PACE program features a comprehensive medical and social service delivery system using an interdisciplinary team approach in an adult day health center that is supplemented by in-home and referral services in accordance with participants' needs. PACE services include, but are not limited to, all Medicare and Medicaid services, including primary care; programs also must provide social work, drugs, nursing facility care, restorative therapies, personal care and supportive services, nutritional counseling, recreational therapy, and meals. The model, which has already substantially moved care outside of institutional walls and into homes, could be an important test bed for more distributed health care approaches.

19) New alternative payment models should encourage the adoption of palliative and hospice care approaches that incorporate distributed care. Community-based **palliative** programs are already in place in parts of the country, and most incorporate telehealth to provide 24/7 support for people

with serious or advanced illness, their families, and their caregivers. Typically, these programs are part of existing large health systems or accountable care organizations, and are funded internally by them—so to spread these programs to smaller organizations, separate revenue streams to support the telehealth component in particular may be needed. As a result, the Centers for Medicare and Medicaid Innovation is now planning a future demonstration project to test a palliative care payment model under Medicare that would be based at least somewhat on two proposals submitted to the Physician-Focused Payment Technical Advisory Committee, or PTAC, from the Coalition to Transform Advanced Care and the American Association of Hospice and Palliative Medicine (AAHPM).[86]

20) Payment models should be developed by public and private sector payers to support **emergency and ambulance services** in caring for patients without transporting them to a hospital if treatment in the emergency department, or hospitalization, can be avoided. In similar initiatives now under way, in such cities as Denver and Englewood, CO, and Albuquerque, NM, payment for on-site treatment, including the use of telehealth links to the hospital, is built-in to contracts. The objective is to save money on ambulance rides and ER visits, and to spare the anxiety and expense of unnecessary ER visits and hospital care for patients. Such EMS-based systems could also be enlisted to provide primary prevention measures for individuals in the community, or to provide training or other steps to assist individuals in self-care.

21) CMS should expand its Health Care Innovation Awards program to specifically test Health Care Without Walls approaches. The innovation awards program funds "compelling new ideas to deliver better health, improved care and lower costs to people enrolled in Medicare, Medicaid and Children's Health Insurance Program (CHIP), particularly those with the highest health care needs." The second round of awards, launched in 2014 and still ongoing, focused in part on "new models of comprehensive care that extend beyond the clinical service delivery setting."[87] The work group recommends that CMS build on this idea if there is a next round of the program.

Knowledge Gaps

There is a plethora of new digital health care technologies coming onto the market, and no health care system can afford, or should procure, all of them. Rigorous efforts should be made to compile evidence on new technologies and the payment models that support their adoption and the move to more distributed forms of care. Specific recommendations in this vein are as follows:

1) Public and private payers should **significantly increase research funding** for health technology assessments on the uses of telemedicine and distributed forms of care, with the specific purpose of assessing quality of care; whether care replacement is taking place; whether savings are being realized; and consumer preferences and perspectives about telehealth care.

2) To the extent possible, such assessments should be part of pilot tests of new technologies in the context of new payment models. Such assessments could take multiple forms, including cost-benefit analysis, cost-utility analysis, cost-effectiveness analysis, cost-minimization analysis, and also budget impact analysis and other forms of economic assessments.

3) In a similar vein, public and private payers, health systems, and others should conduct rigorous, disciplined, and systematic analyses to determine the returns on investment of technological investments. Governmental organizations that should be charged with undertaking these ROI analyses include a CMS, CMMI, and the Agency for Healthcare Research and Quality (AHRQ).

4) The Health Care Without Walls vision embraces the notion that distributed care, by definition, **supports greater patient engagement, empowerment and self-care**. However, those terms can be loose. Research needs to verify that consumers who, for example, routinely engage with providers via email or telemedicine are more engaged and prone to self-care than patients who do not use email or telehealth.

5) More research is needed on the **barriers that FFS payment presents** to the uptake of distributed care. There is a notable lack of understanding at present as to the magnitude and mechanisms of this obstacle. As well, more research is needed on the CPT and claims-based systems of payment for telemedicine to gauge the magnitude and stratification of billing under those codes.

6) The National Quality Forum and other entities that develop, implement, study, and vet patient-focused quality measures should identify new

measures linked to the use of certain tools and technologies and the movement to more distributed care.

Payment and Reimbursement For Health Care Without Walls: Chapter 2 In Brief

1. The role of economic incentives—i.e., payment and reimbursement of health care providers, as well as other actors in the system—is critically important in health care, especially in the United States, with the largest and costliest health care system in the world. The Payment and Reimbursement Work Stream of the Health Care Without Walls initiative considered how payment and reimbursement policies within health care would best support the movement toward more distributed forms of health care, more focus on the upstream drivers of health status, and adoption and use of a broad range of technologies in the new delivery platform.

2. Payment in the U.S. health care system is complex, and technology is paid for in especially complicated and variable ways. In effect, technology is most often paid for indirectly rather than directly. Payment is customarily made to providers for performing services; compensation for the use of any technology effectively incorporated into the determined payment amount. Payment for services may also yield revenues that providers use to make capital investments in technologies that are depreciated over time, as with any other business.

3. Government and public payers also influence the acquisition of technology by health care providers in ways other than direct payment for services. Examples are "certificate of need" programs aimed at regulating construction or creation of new health care facilities or acquisition of technologies such as imaging, as well as government-led efforts to spur acquisition of health information technology over the past two decades.

4. The work stream found that, to date, some payers have been reluctant to pay for approaches and tools, such as telemedicine, at the heart of more distributed health care. Payers have sometimes feared that use of virtual care will be inferior in quality to in person care; that it will add to costs without improving health, or that it will fail to reduce medical expenditures. As a result, the payment and reimbursement work stream sought to incentivize the shift to a more flexible health care system that allows for more

distributed care, and adoption of the technology that would enable it, while avoiding the addition of more cost and complexity to the payment system or further incentivizing delivery of low-value services.

5. The work stream also weighed its recommendations against the backdrop of a U.S. health care system that is transitioning—albeit slowly—from fee-for-service payment to value-based payment. The work stream found that the transition to a more innovative and adaptive system of care in the U.S. would best be achieved via global budgets, capitated systems of payment, and at-risk contracting. However, given the long transition under way from fee-for-service payment to alternative payment models, a "glide path" approach will be needed to greater value-based payment and enhanced use of innovative technologies at the same time.

6. The work stream divided its recommendations into several categories, including recommendations that related to specific new payment incentives for providers; new or expanded federal and state government experimentation with alternative payment models or other novel payment approaches; new incentives aimed at, or to be adopted by, commercial payers and self-insurers; and new financial incentives aimed at patients, individuals, and families themselves.

7. For health care providers and systems, the work stream posited that a variety of new incentives could be created or expanded to incentivize the transition to more distributed modes of health care delivery. These could include episode-based payment or bundles that would enable providers to make use of a range of information and other technologies in the delivery and management of care.

8. With respect to public payers such as Medicare and Medicaid, Congress should direct the Centers for Medicare and Medicaid Services and the Center for Medicare and Medicaid Innovation (CMMI) to expand the volume of demonstrations that included new technology enabled care management and delivery models, to determine whether these models can reduce Medicare and Medicaid expenditures while preserving or enhancing the quality of care. For example, CMS should evaluate the prospect of incorporating distributed care into ongoing dual eligible experiments and payment and delivery reforms, as well as in palliative care and hospice programs. It should also encourage the use and assessment of telehealth and other technology enabled tools in Programs of All-Inclusive Care for the Elderly, or PACE, a unique

capitated managed care benefit for the frail elderly. CMS also should expand its Health Care Innovation Awards program to specifically test Health Care Without Walls approaches.

9. CMS should incentivize Medicare Advantage plans to test new models of care and payment, and to accelerate the transition to global budgets and at-risk contracting for providers. CMS also should expand the existing Medicare Value-Based Insurance Design model[88] to permit MA plans more leeway to test approaches to distributed forms of care coupled with lower cost-sharing for beneficiaries.

10. More states should consider seeking waivers from CMS to emulate a variety of payment experiments in Medicare and Medicaid, including Maryland's all-payer rate setting system; "Section 1115" Medicaid waivers, including Delivery System Reform Incentive Payment (DSRIP) waivers; the Pennsylvania Rural Health Model, under which that state seeks to increase rural Pennsylvanians' access to high-quality care and improve their health, while also reducing the growth of hospital expenditures across payers; and Vermont's All-Payer Accountable Care Organization (ACO) Model. All of these experiments contain inherent incentives to test whether distributed care approaches can substitute for more costly services and improve community-level care.

11. The Health Resources and Services Administration should recommend to Congress, and Congress should enact, federal legislation that permits community health centers to more broadly experiment with distributed care.

12. Congress should create large-scale transformation grants to rural and safety net providers, such as critical access hospitals, to enable them to shift away from their current acute care models and toward becoming community-based health care providers that serve as telehealth facilitators, primary care clinics, substitute observation units for inpatient beds, and provide transport to larger hospitals in more urban settings as needed. The grants would be funded by taxpayers, but could be financed through payment offsets or assumptions about shifts in payment.

13. Other changes should be undertaken by commercial health plans and self-insured employers, or should be instituted in laws and regulations affecting them, to support the shift to more distributed care. For example, commercial payers could be allowed to count their own investments in new

technologies enabling more provision of distributed care as a medical expense for the purposes of the Medical Loss Ratio, rather than as administrative or overhead costs. Self-insured employers could count contributions for health-related technologies that patients used in their homes as part of employer-provided wellness programs, and therefore given tax-free to eligible employees.

14. Patients, consumers, and family caregivers should be incentivized directly to take up the use of technologies that could be clearly linked to improved health outcomes, in part through greater self-care and behavior change. For example, a patient who regularly entered his or her blood glucose levels on an app could receive a small bonus payment—perhaps even via a mobile payment mechanism such as Venmo – once a week's worth of that activity were completed. Payers also could investigate using these types of incentives to enlist patients in primary prevention—e.g., incentivizing young and healthy patients to use fitness trackers or nutrition-oriented apps to maintain good eating and exercise habits and maintain healthy weights. Value-based insurance design models also should be tested, in both commercial insurance and Medicare Advantage plans, as a way to incentivize consumers to choose lower cost providers and modes of care, including telehealth.

15. Rigorous efforts should be made to compile evidence on new technologies and the payment models that support their adoption and the move to more distributed forms of care. Public and private payers should significantly increase research funding for health technology assessments on the uses of telemedicine and distributed forms of care. Returns on investments in technology also should be assessed in a disciplined and systematic way. Such assessments should be part of pilot tests of new technologies in the context of new payment models created by both public and private payers.

16. To ensure value, sets of measures should be developed by the National Quality Forum and other entities to assist in tying payment to outcomes that matter to patients, and for particular use in payment models designed to stimulate the move of care to more distributed settings.

♦ ♦ ♦

End Notes, Chapter 2

[52] "APMs Overview," Quality Payment Program, CMS, accessed May 1, 2018, https://qpp.cms.gov/apms/overview.

[53] Michael Hochman, "Electronic Health Records: a "Quadruple Win, " a "Quadruple Failure," or Simply Time for a Reboot?," *Journal of Internal Medicine* 33, no. 4 (2018): 397-9, DOI: 10.1007/s11606-018-4337-6.

[54] Thomas Beaton, "Competitive Bidding Curbs Medicare Durable Medical Equipment Costs," HealthPayerIntelligence, August 30, 2018, https://healthpayerintelligence.com/news/competitive-bidding-curbs-medicare-durable-medical-equipment-costs.

[55] "Health technology assessment of medical devices", World Health Organization, accessed May 7, 2018, http://apps.who.int/iris/bitstream/10665/44564/1/9789241501361_eng.pdf.

[56] Health Care Payment Learning & Action Network. *Measuring Progress: Adoption of Alternative Payment Models in Commercial, Medicaid, Medicare Advantage, and Fee-for-Service Medicare Programs.* October 30, 2017.

[57] "Bundled Payments for Care Improvement (BPCI) Initiative: General Information," CMS.gov, accessed May 7, 2018, https://innovation.cms.gov/initiatives/bundled-payments/.

[58] "MACRA Basics Advanced Alternative Payment Models (AAPMs)," AAFP, accessed May 7, 2018, https://www.aafp.org/practice-management/payment/medicare-payment/aapms.html.

[59] Jacqueline Belliveau, "PTAC Recommends 2 APMs for Potential MACRA Implementation," RevCycleIntelligence, November 10, 2017, https://revcycleintelligence.com/news/ptac-recommends-2-apms-for-potential-macra-implementation.

[60] Sarah Klein, Martha Hostetter, and Douglas McCarthy, " The Hospital at Home Model: Bringing Hospital-Level Care to the Patient," The Commonwealth Fund, August 22, 2016, http://www.commonwealthfund.org/publications/case-studies/2016/aug/hospital-at-home.

[61] See "Secretary's Response to PTAC commends and recommendations spanning October 2017-May 2018 (PDF)" at https://innovation.cms.gov/initiatives/pfpms/.

[62] Sean Duffy and Thomas H. Lee, "In-Person Health Care as Option B," *The New England Journal of Medicine* 378, no.2(2018): 104-106, DOI: 10.1056/NEJMp1710735.

[63] See https://www.va.gov/COMMUNITYCARE/docs/news/VA_Telehealth_Services.pdf.

[64] Vera Gruessner, "The History of Remote Monitoring, Telemedicine Technology," mHealthIntelligence, November 9, 2015, https://mhealthintelligence.com/news/the-history-of-remote-monitoring-telemedicine-technology.

[65] Breanna Shebel, "Telemedicine is Your New Way to Get Medical Care Without Leaving Home," Mediaplanet, accessed May 7, 2018, http://www.futureofbusinessandtech.com/workplace-wellness/telemedicine-is-your-new-way-to-get-medical-care-without-leaving-home.

[66] See https://obamawhitehouse.archives.gov/sites/default/files/microsites/ostp/PCAST/pcast_independence_tech___aging_report_final_0.pdf.

[67] See http://www.medpac.gov/docs/default-source/reports/chapter-8-telehealth-services-and-the-medicare-program-june-2016-report-.pdf?sfvrsn=0.

[68] "CCM Patient Resources," CMS.gov, accessed May 7, 2018, https://www.cms.gov/About-CMS/Agency-Information/OMH/equity-initiatives/ccm/patient-resources.html.

[69] See https://www.cms.gov/Newsroom/MediaReleaseDatabase/Press-releases/2018-Press-releases-items/2018-07-02-2.html.

[70] "State Telehealth Laws and Reimbursement Policies Report," Center for Connected Health Policy, accessed April 3, 2018, http://www.cchpca.org/state-telehealth-laws-and-reimbursement-policies-report.

[71] J. Scott Ashwood, Ateev Mehrotra, David Cowling, and Lori Uscher-Pines, "Direct-To-Consumer Telehealth May Increase Access to Care But Does Not Decrease Spending," *HealthAffairs* 36, no.3(March 2017):485-491, https://doi.org/10.1377/hlthaff.2016.1130.

[72] Ibid.

[73] J. Scott Ashwood et al., "Retail Clinic Visits for Low-Acuity Conditions Increase Utilization and Spending," *HealthAffairs* 35, no.3(March 2016): 449-55, https://doi.org/10.1377/hlthaff.2015.0995.

[74] See http://www.americantelemed.org/policy-page/state-policy-resource-center.

[75] "Reinventing Rural Health Care," Bipartisan Policy Center, January 2018, https://bipartisanpolicy.org/wp-content/uploads/2018/01/BPC-Health-Reinventing-Rural-Health-Care-1.pdf.

[76] G. Mark Holmes, George H. Pink, Sarah A. Friedman, and Hilda A Howard, "A comparison of rural hospitals with special Medicare payment provisions to urban and rural hospitals paid under prospective payment," August 2010, http://www.shepscenter.unc.edu/rural/pubs/report/FR98.pdf.

[77] Ibid.

[78] See https://oig.hhs.gov/oei/reports/oei-05-12-00080.pdf.

[79] See https://aspe.hhs.gov/system/files/pdf/253406/ProjectSonarSonarMD.pdf.

[80] See https://innovation.cms.gov/Files/x/ptac-projectsonar-letter.pdf.

[81] Mark Lutes and Joel Brill, "CMS Should Invite Innovators To Furnish Technology-Enabled Episodes of Care," Health Affairs Blog, May 14, 2018,https://www.healthaffairs.org/do/10.1377/hblog20180508.688388/full/.

[82] See https://aspe.hhs.gov/system/files/pdf/255906/ProposalPersonalizedRecoveryCare.pdf.

[83] Matt Reynolds, "NHS to start prescribing health apps that help manage conditions," New Scientist, February 13, 2017, https://www.newscientist.com/article/2121164-nhs-to-start-prescribing-health-apps-that-help-manage-conditions/.

[84] "Medicare Advantage Value-Based Insurance Design Model", CMS.gov, accessed May 7, 2018, https://innovation.cms.gov/initiatives/vbid/.

[85] Susan Haber et al., "Evaluation of the Maryland all-payer model: second annual report," March 2018, https://downloads.cms.gov/files/cmmi/md-all-payer-thirdannrpt.pdf.

[86] See https://downloads.cms.gov/files/cmmi/ptac-hhssecresponse-oct17-may18.pdf.

[87] "Health Care Innovation Awards round Two," CMS.gov, accessed May 7, 2018, https://innovation.cms.gov/initiatives/Health-Care-Innovation-Awards/Round-2.html.

[88] "Medicare Advantage Value-Based Insurance Design Model", CMS.gov, accessed May 7, 2018, https://innovation.cms.gov/initiatives/vbid/.

SCENARIO 5:
A YOUNG BOY WITH DEVELOPMENTAL AND PHYSICAL DISABILITIES

LUKE IS A 10-year-old boy with cerebral palsy and an array of developmental, intellectual, and physical disabilities. He has impaired gross and fine motor skills, and is largely confined to a wheelchair; he also has severely impaired speech and substantial intellectual disability. When Luke was diagnosed with these conditions as an infant, his mother, Sophie, quit her job to stay home full-time and care for Luke and his older sister, Mary Ellen. Luke and his family live in a Western state, and Luke is on Medicaid. Sophie is estranged from her husband, Luke's father, and suffers from anxiety and depression.

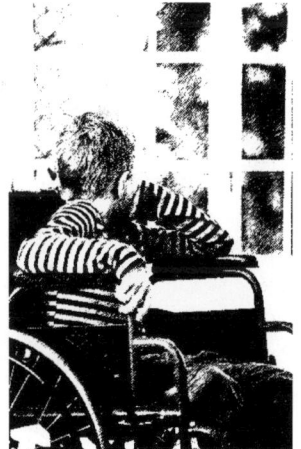

Fifteen percent of American children have a developmental disability, including such conditions as autism and attention deficit and hyperactivity disorder, according to the federal Centers for Disease Control and Prevention. Cerebral palsy is the most common of all childhood disabilities, affecting approximately three live births out of every thousand in the United States. A total of about 764,000 children and adults in the United States currently have cerebral palsy, and about 500,000 children under age of 18 currently have the condition. One in two people with cerebral palsy have an intellectual disability, and 1 in 5 people have a moderate to severe intellectual disability.

Luke has been in an early intervention program for children with developmental disabilities for several years, in which he receives physical, occupational, and speech and language therapy. He needs regular visits with her pediatrician, in part to manage the spasticity associated with her condition, for which he takes the medications baclofen and Botox. Her home is equipped with adaptive equipment, including ramps for her wheelchair. Because transportation is difficult, Luke needs as much of his care as possible to be provided in the home, and his mother needs substantial support to manage her many parental responsibilities.

In the past, the complexities of managing Luke's care have proved overwhelming for Sophie. Her days have been filled with physical visits to various care providers, in anticipation of which she must not only meet Luke's daily care needs, but also help him into his wheelchair and transport him in the family's especially-equipped van. Despite the assistance of a Medicaid case manager, Sophie does not at all feel as if her child's care is at all coordinated. The various clinicians and therapists never speak to each other, and only her pediatrician has an electronic medical record that other care providers cannot access. Sophie is cast in the role of connector and translator, communicating among the various parties about what is going on with Luke, and what her son needs.

In one episode, a social worker came to visit the family on a hot summer day. Sophie reported to the social worker that Luke seemed lethargic, which the social worker chalked up to the high heat. It was only a week later, at a visit with the pediatrician, that the clinician noticed the sluggishness and determined that Luke's medication dose was probably too high. Fortunately, Luke wasn't harmed in the process, but Sophie regretted that she hadn't reported Luke's symptoms to her doctor sooner, and wondered why the social worker hadn't passed along to the physician the observation about Luke's lethargy.

Sophie longs for a care system in which all of these providers could be linked together, and work as a team to help deliver Luke's care across the continuum of her needs. One possibility would be a Medicaid "complex chronic care model," which would incentivize coordination within a care team, and offer comprehensive coverage for virtual visits, technologies, and social supports for Luke and her family. In periodic virtual "visits" with the care team, all members of the team could "see" Luke and speak with her mother about her condition. They could share information, deliberate together about any of Luke's medical or other issues, and in so doing, optimize her care.

Other in-home and virtual supports would help the family enormously and minimize the time and energy that Sophie expends in transporting her son to various appointments. A community health worker could visit periodically and act as the eyes and ears of the pediatrician in between visits. A virtual support group for parents of disabled children could help Sophie cope with the stress of caregiving.

Fortunately, the state in which Luke and his family live have been awarded a federal Innovation Challenge grant to devise new care systems for children with disabilities and complex care needs. Sophie has been appointed to a parents' advisory committee, and looks forward to brainstorming with Medicaid officials and care providers about putting some of her ideas into action.

◆ ◆ ◆

CHAPTER 3: REGULATORY CHANGES TO SUPPORT HEALTH CARE WITHOUT WALLS

U.S. HEALTH CARE is a highly regulated enterprise at the federal, state, and even local level—the paramount reasons for which are the need to ensure a high level of health care quality and safety for consumers and patients, and protection against fraud. As a result, multiple regulatory issues at the federal, state, and local level will pertain to the movement of health care to more distributed settings, thanks to the vast array of regulations that govern the range of personnel who provide health care and who will be using technology; the places and settings in which technology-enabled care is provided; the technology-driven aspects of care that are provided; and technological equipment itself.

There are multiple layers of regulation that govern health care, from the federal Medicare "conditions of participation" regulations that apply to hospitals, to the zoning and other requirements covering health care facilities at the local level. For a wide variety of historical, constitutional, and statutory reasons beyond the scope of this white paper, the U.S. states in particular have wide latitude to regulate how health care is supplied within their borders. State regulations vary greatly among the states, but can govern matters as diverse as the supply of health care facilities through certificate-of-need programs, professional licensure of many health care providers, and benefits provided in health plans (beyond federal minimum requirements). These state regulations can build on federal laws and regulations, and in some instances, can be more rigorous than the federal ones.

Technologies and their use—including many of those employed in health care—also may be subject to regulation by federal agencies, ranging from the Federal Trade Commission and Food and Drug Administration, as well as to certain consumer protection laws and regulations at the state level. Some "wearables" are in fact medical devices that require regulatory approval by the U.S. Food and Drug Administration and some of which will not; software that supplies clinical decision support, much of it supported by artificial or augmented intelligence; technologies such as virtual reality, which create artificial environments to stimulate the senses, and can be used in a variety of ways in health care, including rehabilitation; voice recognition technologies; self-administered laboratory tests, and much more. (A fuller list of these technologies appeared in chapter 1.)

As health care evolves, regulations written for one era of health care pose uncertainties for technology-driven innovations that arise in another. An example is "Hospital at Home," the strategy described in previous chapters of this volume to treat patients who would typically be hospitalized for acute conditions in their homes instead of in the inpatient setting. In some states, such as New York, there has been uncertainty as to whether this approach should be regulated as hospital care, home care, or something altogether different. In New York, where state law prohibited sending nurses from a hospital to a patient's home unless operating under a "home care" license, rather than a "hospital" one, Mount Sinai health system has had to partner with the Visiting Nurse Service of New York, which has such a "home care" license, to conduct nursing visits to patients at home legally.

Another example of a recent innovation that has run into regulatory barriers designed for an earlier era is text messaging. The Centers for Medicare and Medicaid Services, for example, has determined that although text messages have become an important means of communication in health care, health care organizations may only exchange text messages on secure platforms, and clinicians cannot use them to issue orders (which must be executed on computerized physician order entry systems, or by hand).[89] Such restrictions may well be appropriate to protect patients' privacy and to maintain patient safety and security of data. At the same time, however, physicians' use of technologies to communicate with each other, as well as other members of the health care team, is exploding, with little regulation governing its use (beyond privacy restrictions under the Health Insurance Portability and Accountability Act, or HIPAA).

An example is "Figure 1," an online social networking app now widely used by clinicians to send patients' images and brief descriptions of these unnamed and otherwise unidentified patients to each other for clinical recommendations and feedback.[90] In effect a kind of "Instagram" for doctors, the app is now available in more than 100 countries, and allows users either to share information with everyone signed up to use the app, or to communicate directly with specific clinicians via a secure messaging tool built into the app. Because no specific information that would reveal patients' identity is conveyed, the communications have not to date fallen under the purview of the Health Insurance Portability and Accountability Act, or other state privacy statutes. But with millions of users now employing the app worldwide, it is unclear whether any single jurisdiction's regulatory oversight could necessarily keep up.

Regulation of health information

What's more, because much of health care now depends on exchanges of digital information, specific areas of regulation not unique to health care, but more generally applicable to information in general, now play an important role. For example, the Federal Communications Commission regulates the broadband channels on which information, including health information, flows. Under various federal and state laws, strict privacy protections apply to the exchange of so-called protected health information. The Federal Trade Commission enforces a range of sector-specific privacy laws, as well as the Federal Trade Commission Act's broad prohibition against "unfair or deceptive acts" or practices, all of which can apply to the exchange of data from wearable monitors, for example.

A further complexity is that, in US health care, regulation is often very closely tied to payment. Certain regulations will pertain to health care facilities or procedures based on whether they can be reimbursed or paid for based on billing codes, Medicare conditions of participation, and the like. This particular duality—regulation tied to payment—creates special problems in the context of virtual care that is cutting across older care, reimbursement, and regulatory silos.

Finally, in an increasingly global marketplace for many aspects of health care, such as drugs and devices, differences in regulation among countries also affect health care. For example, the European Union (E.U.) regulates information privacy and security very differently from the US and according to stricter overall standards, but health care device manufacturers must observe the E.U. regulations in this sphere in order to sell their devices in Europe, and other information companies have had to amend their policies to accommodate users in the E.U. An important issue for the U.S.

digital health data sector is whether there will be future efforts to harmonize U.S. and European Union regulations, and if not, what the implications will be for consumers, technology producers, product design, sales, and profitability.

Goals of Regulatory Work Stream

The Regulatory Work Stream of the Health Care Without Walls initiative was charged with the following objectives:

Taking into account the vision developed by the Technology Work Stream as to what the delivery of health care could look like in 2025, the work stream should highlight the regulatory areas that will come into play as a more distributed system evolves. Examples include governmental approval of digital health products and devices; regulations governing privacy, security, and health information retention; and health professional licensure and scope of practice, among others.

The work stream was also charged with recommending actions that should be taken by a range of relevant actors to support the evolution of Health Care Without Walls, including the U.S. Congress and state legislatures, and the pertinent regulatory agencies at the federal and state level, such as the Food and Drug Administration; the Centers for Medicare and Medicaid Services; the Office of the National Coordinator of Health Information Technology; the Federal Communications Commission; the Federal Trade Commission; and the Department of Health and Human Services Office of Civil Rights; state departments of health and other agencies that regulate hospitals, pharmacies, home health agencies, health care facilities, and other aspects of health care delivery; and state boards governing health professional licensure.

Finally, the Regulatory Work Stream was asked to pose issues that other work streams should tackle, and recommendations they should make, to support the Health Care Without Walls vision, and to identify any critical research gaps about regulation that should be filled in the interests of moving to a more distributed care system.

Policy Objectives

Participants in the Health Care Without Walls Regulatory Work Stream said that they believed that an overall policy goal should be to produce a regulatory framework at the federal and state levels that would support evolution of a more distributed care system, and deliver the benefits of a more accessible, timely, convenient, and lower cost health care system while preserving or advancing quality and safety. For the time being, they observed, specific regulatory obstacles are actually impeding the development of Health Care Without Walls in a variety of ways.

A useful framework that the work stream adopted was to examine regulation in four domains: regulation over people, places, processes, and products. In each domain lie obstacles to development of a more distributed system.

Regulation over People and Their Practice

Regulation of "people"—the professionals and personnel operating within health care—is for the most part state-based through licensure and related requirements. Licensure allows professionals, such as physicians, to practice certain acts and procedures within health care and within the state. Practice and licensure rules vary greatly among states; for example, scope of practice legislation imposes very different restrictions on the types of activities that different licensed professionals can engage in (see the Work Force chapter for more discussion of this issue). The application of state licensure to telemedicine and telehealth, however, is potentially even more complicated. Indeed, "No two states are alike in how telehealth is defined or regulated," asserts a 2017 report by the Center for Connected Health Policy.[91]

Each state has its own licensure qualifications and laws pertaining to the practice of medicine within the state that bear on the practice of telehealth or telemedicine. Most states require that a physician or other health care professional be licensed in the state where their patient is located, and some states require a physical visit prior to usage of telemedicine and/or prescribing over the internet. A few states issue and require specific licenses for the practice of telehealth. In general, state-based licensure has hindered the practice of telemedicine across state lines. Although several interstate compacts have been created to expedite licensure in multiple states for physicians, nurses, and midlevel health care providers, in some instances these arrangements are developing slowly and are not actually encouraging virtual care. For example, the interstate compact sponsored by the National Association of State Medical Boards only smooths the path for a physician licensed in one state to acquire an additional license in a new state in order to practice telemedicine into that state; multiple state licenses are still required. Some states are considering legislation specifically to allow physicians with valid licenses in other states to practice telemedicine on patients within the state, but as of the publication of this report, no states have approved that arrangement.

Nursing has taken a different approach that is more supportive of telemedicine. The Nurse Licensure Compact is an interstate compact that allows a nurse to have one multistate license (in his or her state of residency) and to practice in other states (both physically and electronically), subject to each state's practice laws and regulation. As of 2018, 25 states have signed on.

In general, the work stream concluded, this thicket of licensure-based regulation over telehealth and telemedicine is impractical, and ill serves the public as well as health professionals. The work stream's recommendations to evolve new licensure systems are contained below. Underserved areas of the country in particular stand to benefit from an expansion of licensure standards governing telehealth. Work stream participants pointed to the example of the Veterans Health Administration. Currently, VA providers can waive state licensing requirements if both the physician and the patient are in a federally owned facility; as a result, telehealth consultations within the VA system are increasingly common.

But with the development of a new mobile app, the VA now also wants to reach veterans in their homes to expand access to mental health services, and to make it easier for those with limited mobility to get necessary medical care. For example, a pilot VA program is currently administering psychotherapy and related services by telehealth to rural veterans suffering from post-traumatic stress disorder; psychotherapy is delivered by interactive video from a VA medical center to one of 12 clinics across the nation, or directly to the veteran's home, by off-site psychiatrists and psychologists. Legislation has now passed both the House (HR 2123) and Senate (S 925) to allow any VA licensed health care professional to practice telemedicine at any location in any state, regardless of where the professional or patient is based. However, as of publication of this report, slight differences between the bills have not yet been reconciled and the provisions have not yet been enacted into law.

Regulation over Places

Regulation of "places," or settings in which health care is provided, and the care that is provided within them, is effectively spread across the federal and state levels. On the federal level, Medicare has "conditions of participation" or "conditions for coverage"—the minimum health and safety standards that providers and suppliers of health services must meet to qualify for Medicare certification and reimbursement. An independent, not-for-profit organization, The Joint Commission, also accredits and certifies nearly 21,000 health care organizations and programs in the United States. For their part, states regulate health care facilities in a variety of ways. Depending on the state, and the type of facility, multiple agencies, departments, boards, bureaus, and commissions may have regulatory authority in the form of various licensure, accreditation, and other requirements.

Existing regulations and structures are proving to be challenging in some instances as health care moves outside of traditional institutions and facilities. For example, it is unclear in some states, such as New York, whether hospital-at-home programs can send nurses to patients' homes as part of that hospital license, or whether such programs must be regulated as home-care agencies—even though the hospital-at-home approach technically is not providing what would normally be considered home health care. In a recent report, "Putting Patients First," the New York State Health Department reported that it recognized the fundamental problem: "The rapid pace of health care innovation and reform has outpaced the ability of New York State's regulatory structure to adapt, resulting in a regulatory landscape that can be complex and outdated."[92] As noted previously, the Mount Sinai system has elected to deal with the ambiguity in state regulation by forging a partnership with the Visiting Nurse Service of New York, a licenses home care provider, to handle the dispatch of nurses to homes.

How might regulatory accommodations be made to accommodate health care delivery in novel settings on something other than a state-by-state basis? One possibility, advanced as a recommendation below, could be devising a model statute that could be adopted separately by states. Such a statue would create a new category of appropriate licensure and oversight of health care practice outside of facilities, or of care transcending facilities, and adopt through that process nationwide standards for what constitutes safe, efficacious, cost-effective health care in untraditional, diverse, or even virtual settings.

Under such an approach, care would not be defined by the site—"home" or "hospital"—but rather by the diagnosis and acuity of the patient. Thus, in addition to its hospital license, institutions such as Mount Sinai could obtain an "acute care license" allowing it to care for specified types of patients in multiple settings—at home, via telehealth, or whatever it deemed appropriate. Another approach that the work stream discussed would be creation of model state legislation that would empower state departments of health, or other agencies that license health care facilities and service providers to exercise flexibility in the case where a provider already in possession of a hospital license sought to provide non-hospital services, such as home-based care, that was consistent with hospital care and was not marketed or promoted as a stand-alone service.

The work stream pointed to a model that is evolving for regulating a program or type of care, irrespective of place, as in the Diabetes Prevention Program (DPP) interventions now accredited by the Centers for Disease Control and Prevention and covered under the Medicare program.[93] This lifestyle change program, aimed at people who have pre-diabetes that could evolve to full-blown diabetes emphasizes self-monitoring and problem-solving to encourage healthy eating, physical activity, and weight loss; provides for coach feedback; includes participant materials to support program goals; and calls for participant weigh-ins to track progress. To be accredited by CDC and eligible for Medicare reimbursement, DPP programs must include specific clinical content and adhere to quality and outcome standards that apply across all settings, whether provided in person or virtually via secure, digital communications. Such accreditation of health care programs independent of setting could be one direction in which state regulation over health care "places" also could evolve.

Regulation over Processes

There is a broad swath of federal law and regulation that applies to processes within health care, ranging from coding standards to Stark laws and the Anti-Kickback statute. The Stark laws prohibit physician self-referral, or a referral by a physician of a Medicare or Medicaid patient to an entity providing designated health services if the physician or an immediate family member has a financial relationship with that entity. The federal **Anti-Kickback Statute** is a criminal **statute** that prohibits the exchange or offer to exchange, of anything of value, in an effort to induce or reward the referral of federal health care program business.

Another process that is closely regulated by the federal government and by states is prescription of controlled substances. Under the federal Ryan Haight Act, no controlled substance may be delivered, distributed, or dispensed by means of the internet (which, for all practical purposes, includes telemedicine technologies) without a valid prescription.[94]

According to this article, "a valid prescription is one that is issued for a legitimate medical purpose in the usual course of professional practice by: 1) a practitioner who has conducted at least one in-person medical evaluation of the patient; or 2) a covering practitioner. An "in-person medical evaluation" means a medical evaluation that is conducted with the patient in the physical presence of the prescribing practitioner. Under the Ryan Haight Act, it is a violation of the <u>federal Controlled Substances Act</u>[95] for a practitioner to issue a prescription for a controlled substance by means of the Internet without having conducted at least one in-person medical evaluation, except in certain specified circumstances.

Although the law provides for an exception to the in-person evaluation requirement when a provider is engaged in the practice of telemedicine, the provider must maintain a DEA registration at each site where a patient is located. This requirement compels providers engaged in telemedicine or telehealth to maintain multiple DEA registrations, which can be costly and administratively burdensome. Such restrictions particularly affect specialties that couple chronic disease management with pharmacotherapy, such as telepsychiatry, substance abuse/recovery, endocrinology, hormone replacement therapy, and medical weight loss.

In 2016, DEA announced plans to issue a new rule to adopt a nationwide DEA registration that would allow clinicians to use telemedicine to prescribe controlled substances in any state under a single registration. The work stream encouraged DEA to move forward and promulgate this program.

Regulation over Products

The vast array of products, technologies, and equipment employed in the virtual delivery of health care are regulated in multiple ways by both the federal government and the states. Regulation of products considered to be medical devices occurs mainly at the federal level, and is evolving, but slowly, and leaves a number of gray areas of regulation as technology evolves. In recent years, however, the U.S. Food and Drug Administration has taken an increasingly proactive stance in regulation of digital health—categories such as mobile health (mHealth), health information technology (IT), wearable devices, telehealth and telemedicine, and aspects of personalized medicine. The FDA's Center for Devices and Radiological Health introduced a Digital Health Innovation Action Plan in 2017 with the goal of fostering innovation while focusing the agency's attention and oversight on higher-risk products. As the FDA put it in the Action Plan, released in 2017:

"We focused our oversight on mobile medical apps to only those that present higher risk to patients, while choosing not to enforce compliance for lower-risk mobile apps…We chose not to focus our oversight on products that only promote general wellness."[96]

In November 2017, FDA also announced the first of a series of pilots to begin establishing a Digital Health Software Precertification (Pre-Cert) Program. The intent is to modernize the regulatory approval process for the software design and programming that underpins many digital health devices. This proposed voluntary program to "pre-certify" companies that perform high-quality software design and testing will replace the need for these developers to file premarket submissions to the FDA for approval, and in some cases will allow for faster review of marketing applications.

The Regulatory Work Stream applauded these moves by the FDA, and was especially enthusiastic about the Pre-Cert program. At the same time, work stream participants noted a number of gray areas and lack of clarity on which types of devices and technologies need to be approved, and by whom. For example, with certain novel technologies, there are at times disagreement within FDA when these technologies straddle the areas of software and diagnostics, and are thus potentially subject to review by the Office of Device Evaluation, which regulates certain medical software apps, and the office of In Vitro Diagnostics, which regulates diagnostics.

Separate and apart from digital health, there is also a special set of issues around diagnostics and lab tests and differences in regulation for FDA-approved versus lab-based tests that are "waived" under the Clinical Laboratory Improvement Amendments of 1988 (CLIA). Ambiguity in this area could create confusion in the regulation of self-administered lab tests and "point of care" diagnostics, which are likely to be other hallmarks of Health Care Without Walls systems. As of the date of publication of this report, the FDA is in the process of releasing new guidance in this arena, which could expand the number of "waived" tests and offer further clarification.

Clinical Decision Support

There are also various regulatory issues pertaining to clinical decision support software, as well as the growing functions of machine learning, artificial intelligence, and augmented intelligence that are increasingly used in support of clinical practice. The FDA is regulating in this area because it has broad authority over ensuring that any claims made in a product label are clinically safe—that is, that any recommendations produced by the CDS software (and the machine learning algorithms and artificial intelligence that develops the recommendation) are not harmful to patients. Meanwhile, the Federal Trade Commission also has a role, which is ensuring that products sold to or used by consumers are not harmful, and that claims about them are not false or misleading (e.g., if a manufacturer makes claims about data encryption on its device that turn out not to be true). What's more, states, with their own independent powers to protect consumers, are also taking action and becoming involved in regulating CDS and other systems under consumer protection statutes.

The FDA issued its clinical decision support regulatory guidance in December 2017 after a six-year process, and essentially embraced the regulatory framework set forth in the 21st Century Cures Act. Under the FDA's approach, the agency will not require regulatory approval of software if any recommendations that the software makes are to be independently reviewed by and/or acted upon by physicians, or other learned intermediaries. However, some analysts have raised concerns that the FDA guidance fails to consider the next generation of medical software that integrates machine learning and artificial intelligence.[97]

The Clinical Decision Support Coalition, a private group of individuals and organizations who want to make or use software, including artificial intelligence, to improve the quality of health care (see www.cdscoalition.org) has finalized its own set of guidelines to provide a pathway for "medium-risk" software that uses complex algorithms to proceed without going through FDA approval (e.g., a software tool that predicts the likelihood of a migraine). Still, concerns remain that no bright line has been drawn over regulating "higher-risk" software. For example, a software tool that recommends a specific chemotherapy treatment for a patient could be considered "higher risk" because its AI-enabled recommendations could amount to life-or-death decisions, if that recommendation were not reviewed by a physician first.[98]

Further discussion of the issue of regulation of artificial intelligence is below, under the heading "Regulation of Artificial Intelligence."

Regulation over Health Information Privacy, Security, and Data Exchange

Information privacy and security are separate but related issues, since the security of data is directly related to the degree to which it is held safely and accords privacy for the individual person, or group of people, to whom the data relate. Even seemingly innocuous data exposed and used thoughtlessly can disclose private health information or other important confidential information. In recent years, a number of incidents have occurred in which private health information, including protected health information (PHI) has been exposed or hacked;[99] in other episodes, health insurers' records also have been exposed, as was the case in a massive hack of Anthem in 2015 likely to have been instigated by a foreign government. With more consumer health information now contained in wearables and apps, and amid recent disclosures of misuse of data compiled by Facebook, concerns about the privacy, security, and potential misuse of this information have only grown.

A recent episode illustrates this development vividly. In early 2018, an Australian university analyst discovered that a publicly available activity map created by the fitness tracking app Strava showed the fitness routes (for jogging, cycling, etc.) of soldiers and other agents in sensitive locations, including American bases in Afghanistan and Syria, the UK's Mount Pleasant airbase in the Falkland Islands, and suspected CIA base in Somalia. Although no data were released that were specifically pegged to identified people (no names were released, for example) the data had enough context to make it reasonably possible to identify people and their locations. As a result, the US Central Command subsequently announced that it would refine its "privacy" policies based on the reality that apps such as these, mapping people's exercise habits, could pose security risks for forces around the world.[100]

Another hypothetical possibility could arise based on a reported incident in 2018 in which the Alexa app on an Amazon Echo device inadvertently recorded a conversation between individuals and then sent the recording to a third party.[101] Specifically, as the couple was having a discussion, the app was somehow triggered to make the recording without the couple knowing it, and then was triggered to search the couple's list of contacts and send the recording to one of the husband's employees. According to an account in The Washington Post, Amazon said it was "evaluating options to make this case even less likely," but it would not be a stretch to contemplate the dangers of a similar episode involving inadvertent transmission of private health information—for example, a recording of an exchange between a patient and a home care provider about a sensitive health matter.

As more health care is supplied outside traditional health care systems and settings, multiple regulatory issues will arise in the realms of health information privacy and security. Many of them will stem from a growing bifurcation in regulation over so-called protected health information (PHI), which is governed by the federal HIPAA statute and multiple state statutes, and the ever-larger amount of health information that is being collected outside the HIPAA context, such as from wearables. Others will come from a complex overlay of regulatory regimes over information security.

For example, there is overlap and confusion among the Office of Civil Rights at the Department of Health and Human Services, which oversees the federal Health Insurance Portability and Accountability Act, (HIPAA), as described further below; the FDA, which oversees data security and integrity from the standpoint over the way a device operates, not over any information exchange directly; the U.S. Federal Trade Commission, the primary federal consumer protection agency, which has been the principal federal regulator of online privacy practices, primarily through enforcement actions under consumer protection law; and the Federal Communications Commission, which in 2016 began to assert authority to regulate the privacy practices of broadband Internet providers.[102]

Privacy

The U.S. legal framework over health care privacy is a complex combination of statutory, and regulatory law at the federal and state levels. At the federal level, regulations created under HIPAA govern the privacy and security of PHI—individually identifiable health information—that is created or collected by a Covered Entity (CE), defined as a health plan, health care clearinghouse, or health care provider (physician's office, clinic, hospital, pharmacy, nursing home, or other) that electronically transmits any health information.

What's more, if a covered entity engages a so-called Business Associate (BA) to help it carry out its health care activities and functions, the covered entity must have a written contract or other arrangement with the business associate that establishes specifically what the business associate has been engaged to do and requires the business associate to comply with HIPAA requirements to protect the privacy and security of protected health information. (A "business associate" is a person or entity that performs certain functions or activities that involve the use or disclosure of protected health information on behalf of, or provides services to, a covered entity.)

Most states also have enacted their own laws, regulations, and standards about the use, collection, and disclosure of health information. In many instances these state statutes are more protective of privacy than federal law. The differences between federal and state laws pertaining to privacy of health information have long posed challenges for both the health care system and for technology developers. The Office of the National Coordinator for Health Information Technology (ONC), the federal agency charged with helping to establish frameworks for electronic disclosure of health information, has an entire section of its website devoted to this problem (see, for example, https://www.healthit.gov/topic/privacy-security-and-hipaa/health-it-privacy-and-security-resources-providers). Even for an intervention as comparatively widespread as tele-psychiatry, it is unclear which privacy laws govern the exchange: Those where the psychiatrist is located or those where the patient is located, assuming that the laws are different in each place.

Work stream members stressed that it is important for consumers and patients to trust that their protected health information will remain private and secure. To that end, the federal government has recently attempted to clarify what is permissible in the realm of exchanging protected health information without obtaining patients' consent, by spelling out the uses for which it is permissible to transfer such information from a covered entity to another covered entity or business associate.[103] Generally, a business associate or covered entity under HIPAA can transfer protected health information for the purposes of payment, health care treatment, or operations, but all other transfers require consent. An example cited by ONC, of an exchange of PHI that would be permissible without obtaining patients' consent, would be when a given health care provider seeks to share information with an individual's health plan about a patient's need to participate in a diabetes management program. In such a case, the ONC says, the provider should disclose that the exchange of protected health information is necessary for the diabetes management program to be effective.

At the same time, there is growing ambiguity over the fact that much of the health information now being collected about patients and consumers falls outside of the HIPAA/PHI context and outside of covered entities. For example, data collected by Fitbit or a remote sensor in one's home is not a CE and is not governed by HIPAA. It is, however, "consumer information" that is governed by the Federal Trade Commission, and in essence is subject to the FTC's fair information practice principles, which are guidelines for maintaining privacy-friendly, consumer-oriented data collection practices.

These principles and guidelines are far less protective of information security and privacy than HIPAA, and are not enforceable by law. However, many companies adhere to them through self-regulation – for example, by issuing, and requiring consumers to accept, lengthy privacy policies as a condition of using a company's equipment, web site, or other capability. The FTC does evaluate these self-regulation practices, provides guidance for industry in developing information practices, and uses its authority under the FTC Act to enforce promises made by corporations in their privacy policies."[104]

Although not considered protected health information governed by HIPAA, much of this type of information is considered to be "personally Identifiable Information," or data that could potentially identify a specific individual. Collection, use, and distribution of such personally identifiable information is usually governed by state law (nearly all states and the District of Columbia have regulations governing the general use and release of personally identifiable information without patients' consent, although the provisions governing release of such data vary by state.)[105]

What's more, the differences among states, in terms of regulation of data and information privacy, appears to be increasing. In June 2018, for example, both houses of the California legislature unanimously adopted the California Consumer Privacy Act of 2018 (AB 375),[106] the nation's strictest data privacy law to date. Effective in 2020, the law will grant consumers the right to request all information that businesses have collected on them; the right to object to having their data sold; the right to receive their data in a portable format; and the right to ask businesses to delete their personal data. Much will now have to be fleshed out through regulation, but at minimum, entities that compile all forms of health information may now be faced with the difficulties of complying with one very strict set of regulations in California that may or may not be in place in all the other U.S. states.

Notwithstanding the variety of laws and regulations governing such "personally identifiable information" that falls outside the "protected health information" context, there are broad concerns that such information is not sufficiently private or secure for consumers, and thus is subject to potential misuse. A Federal Trade Commission study of 12 health-related mobile apps, for example, found that they transmitted information about such sensitive health conditions as pregnancy, as well as gender and ovulation, to 76 third parties such as ad networks and analytics firms.[107] It is considered likely by legal experts that the FTC could assert its authority to enforce actions against a wearable manufacturer that failed to prevent unauthorized transfers of sensitive information, and private companies have also taken steps to mitigate risks in the way they design their products, and by informing users about their privacy policies.

Nonetheless, the ambiguities and absence of clear laws and regulations around such information gathering and transfer capabilities raise concerns. Not only are consumers at least somewhat unprotected, but businesses seeking to collect or use such data also face the ambiguity as well. "It's very fuzzy right now and it's holding back many organizations from doing that remote patient care, because they're not sure who can, and how would they secure (the data collected)," a Regulatory Work Stream participant noted. "We need something that clarifies, gives clear direction as to…who gets to do what, and up to what limit, and what requirements are around that type of care stakeholder."

Regulatory Work Stream participants noted other concerns as well. There is no clear guidance around "collateral surveillance" from remote monitoring devices, for example, in the home. If patients opt in to such a service, what protections would or should be accorded to someone else who has entered the home and has not opted in to any monitoring agreement?

Others raised the example of the first digitally coded pill, Abilify MyCite, a drug with a sensor that is activated by stomach fluids, and that sends a signal to a patch worn by the patient and notifies a smartphone app that the medication (in this case, the psychiatric medicine Abilify) has been taken. Even assuming that a patient is fully aware of the digital signaling technology, in how much detail do issues like transmission security for the signal need to be disclosed before treatment begins? What is a fair way to warn patients that anyone whom they allow to use their cell phone might gain access to the information about this psychiatric medicine?

A core issue is whether HIPAA should be expanded to cover more health-related information that is not currently deemed protected health information, or, in the absence of such an action, what if any other laws and regulations on data collection, privacy and security should apply. There are also emerging global regulatory frameworks that will govern all internet-based data transfer practices, including those that pertain to health information, such as the European Union's General Data Protection Regulation (GDPR), which went into effect in May 2018. The GDPR is designed to give individuals better control over their personal data and establish one single set of data protection rules across Europe. It also imposes strict rules on entities hosting and processing the data of EU citizens anywhere in the world. In addition, under the European Union-United States Privacy Shield, U.S. companies must commit to robust obligations regarding the processing of any personal data from Europe.

In general, the EU's protection of privacy, including personally identifiable medical information, means that digital health information within the EU will be regulated the same everywhere, no matter where it is collected, by what means it is collected, or who collects it, and that the collection of data and information about all EU citizens everywhere must be held to the same standard. A key part of the GDPR requires consent to be given by the individual whose data is held, and allows that individual to withdraw consent at any time and compel the data to be erased. Although far stricter than what is required in the United States, the simplicity and clarity of this regulatory framework may help Europe move health care "beyond walls" faster than will be possible in the United States. Work stream participants recognized the difficulty of achieving such a common standard in the United States, but argued that the approach of a common data privacy and security framework across the states should be on the table for discussion.

Work stream participants recognized the difficulty of achieving such a common standard in the United States, and noted that the urgency of having that discussion may have only become greater since California enacted the nation's strictest data privacy law in June 2018, as discussed above. Otherwise, all holders of health data and information, whether "protected health information" or not, may have no choice but to play by one set of rules in California and other sets of rules in every other U.S. state—or else effectively comply with California's rules as the new de facto national standard. Since much of that statute will need to be fleshed out with regulation, there will be considerable uncertainty in this arena for some time to come.

Digital health device and systems developers note that uncertainties, ambiguities, and confusion in these areas militate against new product and service development, and therefore could impede evolution of Health Care Without Walls approaches. Undoubtedly much more thought leadership and research in this arena would be helpful. A rigorous academic research agenda should be developed that focuses on, for example, the economics of privacy and security, especially in the health area. The work stream also recommended that Congress convene hearings on the topic of developing a common privacy and security framework around health information and data of all types that can protect consumers and still allow for considerable innovation in health care.

Regulation of Artificial Intelligence

A growing area of discussion is the prospect of specific regulation of artificial intelligence—computer systems that are able to mimic functions that humans associated with other human minds, and therefore are able to perform tasks that normally require human intelligence, such as visual perception, speech and pattern recognition, decision-making, and translation between languages. Artificial intelligence technologies include machine learning, cognitive computing, and augmented intelligence, among others, and the range as likely to expand in the future. As has been noted, "as machines become increasingly capable, tasks considered as requiring 'intelligence' are often removed from the definition," and the resulting technology ceases to be described as artificial intelligence (see https://en.wikipedia.org/wiki/Artificial_intelligence).

As noted in the Technology section of this report, there are potentially innumerable applications of artificial intelligence to the health care sphere, from autonomous vehicles for use in health care that will be equipped with remote sensors to monitor patients' symptoms, to imaging systems that use algorithms to provide diagnostic information about certain types of cancers. It is likely that many of these applications will play a major role in future distributed health care systems, and in so doing, create many new capabilities that will provide major benefits for patients. Yet amid great uncertainties as to how far overall AI technologies will develop, and fears that some applications may prove harmful or be used toward harmful ends, there are growing calls to regulate artificial intelligence, along with equally vocal calls to resist such regulation. Tesla CEO Elon Musk, for example, advised a meeting of the bipartisan National Governors Association in July 2017 that artificial intelligence posed an "existential threat" to human civilization and that proactive regulation of the field was required.

Taking a different tack, an October 2016 report released by the National Science and Technology Council and the White House Office of Science and Technology Policy, "Preparing for the Future of Artificial Intelligence,"[108] noted that the general consensus of those who had responded to a federal request for information on the topic was that "broad regulation of AI research or practice would be inadvisable at this time." The report further notes that if a perceived AI risk "falls within the bounds of an existing regulatory regime, the policy discussion should start by considering whether the existing regulations already adequately address the risk, or whether they need to be adapted to the addition of AI."

On this point, it is clear that federal agencies are now trying to sort out how existing laws and regulation should apply to AI-based health care products and services. For example, as noted above, the Food and Drug Administration has already begun to signal how it will approach regulation of certain AI technologies as devices through guidance documents issued in late 2017. In draft guidance[109] on the regulation of clinical decision support software (defined as software that is intended to provide decision support for the diagnosis, treatment, prevention, cure, or mitigation of diseases or other conditions), FDA spelled out which types of decision support software functionalities do or do not meet the definition of a device, and therefore will or will not be a focus of FDA regulatory oversight. Pointing to language in the 21st Century Cures Act, which exempted from FDA regulation health software "intended for use to analyze information to provide patient-specific recommended options to consider in the prevention, diagnosis, treatment, cure, or mitigation of a particular disease or condition," the guidance in effect suggests that FDA will not regulate as a device capabilities such as IBM Watson, a machine learning or cognitive computing system.

More details on FDA involvement in AI regulation are contained in the December 2017 JASON report by the MITRE Corporation.[110] It notes that the FDA has closely followed the international development of software in medical devices (SiMD) and software as a medical device, both of which can be applications of AI. The FDA has chaired an International Medical Device Regulators forum on SiMD and SaMD, and issued its report for public comment.[111] The FDA plans to use that input to guide its new development of regulation for SiMD and SaMD and to be responsive to new policies under the 21st Century Cures Act.

Meanwhile, the Clinical Decision Support Coalition has released (PDF) draft voluntary guidelines[112] for software developers to ensure that clinical decision support software remains as a support tool for clinicians—not a substitute for human judgment. An important element of these guidelines is transparency to users about the software's workings and capabilities—for example, "Does the software provide enough information for the user to understand and be able to evaluate the clinical basis for the software recommendation?" More broadly, many experts have called for a framework for holding accountable the algorithms used in artificial intelligence applications—for example, to enable them to be discoverable and auditable by all users.[113] As the "Principles for Accountable Algorithms and a Social Impact Statement for Algorithms" developed by the voluntary organization for Fairness, Accountability, and Transparency in Machine Learning state, "There is always a human ultimately responsible for decisions made or informed by an algorithm. 'The algorithm did it' is not an acceptable excuse if algorithmic systems make mistakes or have undesired consequences, including from machine-learning [or artificial intelligence] processes."

As evidence that such a set of accountability principles is necessary, experts point to various instances in which non-transparent algorithms resulted in decisions or actions that harmed individuals in one way or another. For example, algorithms were employed by the states of Arkansas and Idaho to make decisions about home care benefits that caused a cutback in home care benefits.[114] In the Idaho case, a resulting lawsuit showed that the algorithm was based on flawed data. As an article reporting on these instances notes, "Even if the details of the algorithms are accessible, which isn't always the case, they're often beyond the understanding even of the people using them, raising questions about what transparency means in an automated age, and concerns about people's ability to contest decisions made by machines."[115]

Amid concerns about the need to balance ongoing innovation in health care with appropriate safeguards, multiple organizations are now making policy pronouncements and issuing other guidance to signal specific concerns. For example, in June 2018, the American Medical Association adopted its first policy on "augmented intelligence," citing its intent to "Explore the legal implications of health care AI, such as issues of liability or intellectual property, and advocate for appropriate professional and governmental oversight for safe, effective, and equitable use of and access to health care AI."[116]

The Regulatory Work Stream expressed support for these types of voluntary efforts to raise awareness about the risks inherent in over-reliance on artificial intelligence, and to hold industry accountable for self-regulation along these lines as the field evolves. These self-regulatory efforts should clearly focus on transparency and accountability of algorithmic functions, as well as user involvement in AI design. The work stream also expressed agreement with the recommendation of the 2016 Obama Administration report on artificial intelligence that federal agencies should be able to "draw on appropriate technical expertise at the senior level when setting regulatory policy for AI enabled products." This statement clearly implies that federal as well as state agencies will need to beef up their internal technical capabilities to understand the range of issues that may arise and, if necessary, to take appropriate regulatory action.

Broadband Internet Access

Broadband technologies are integral to a system of Health Care Without Walls, and yet according to the Organization of Economic Cooperation and Development, the United States has costlier and lower quality broadband than other countries, and trails most other highly developed countries in the percentage of people with broadband subscriptions.[117] In addition, "the rate of broadband deployment in urban and suburban and high-income areas is outpacing deployment in rural and low-income areas[118] (see Congressional Research Service report). Roughly speaking, as of 2014, the Federal Communications Commission calculated that approximately 10 percent of Americans lacked access to broadband operating at "minimum broadband benchmark speed" of 25 megabits per second for downloads and 3 megabits per second uploads. In rural areas, approximately 39 percent of residents lacked such access. As of 2013, an estimated 73.4 percent of American households had paid broadband subscription. An issue is what to do about this "digital divide," either from a regulatory or federal assistance standpoint.

In January 2017, FCC chairman Ajit Pai formed a new federal advisory committee, the Broadband Deployment Advisory Committee, to provide advice and recommendations for the FCC on how to accelerate the deployment of broadband by reducing and/or removing regulatory barriers to infrastructure investment. However, it is not clear what the committee has accomplished, and in general, regulatory frameworks and policies are not advancing as quickly as technology. The Senate Broadband Caucus, led by Sens. Amy Klobuchar (D-MN), Shelley Moore Capito (R-WV), Angus King (Independent-ME), John Boozman (R-Ark.), and Heidi Heitkamp (D-ND), has made rural broadband one of its highest priorities. FCC and the National

Cancer Institute have also reached an MOU over extending connected care access to rural cancer patients in Appalachia.[119] In July 2018, FCC Commissioner Brendan Carr announced that the agency would seek to establish a new $100 million "Connected Care Pilot Program" for low-income patients, including those eligible for Medicaid or veterans receiving cost-free medical care. The measure would require a congressional appropriation, and if authorized, Carr said, would support "a limited number of projects over a two- or three-year period with controls in place to measure and verify the benefits, costs, and savings associated with connected care."[120]

The Senate Broadband Caucus has argued that stand-alone funding for rural broadband deployment should be part of any large-scale infrastructure plan enacted by Congress and the executive branch, and in 2017, the Trump administration signaled it would make expansion of broadband to rural areas a part of its much-discussed $1 trillion package of public and private sector infrastructure investment. That package included $25 billion for that purpose, amid estimates that extending broadband to all underserved areas of the country would cost closer to $80 billion. As of the publication of this report, no broad infrastructure plan has advanced in Congress.

Yet as the CRS report cited above notes, "a wide variety of policy instruments are available to policymakers" to spur broadband development, including reforming universal service requirements, reducing regulatory barriers to broadband deployment, and clarifying spectrum policy to spur rollout of wireless broadband services." Other approaches could include grants and loans to towns or rural cooperatives; tax credits to incentivize private companies to expand into underserved areas; and "reverse auctions," in which internet service providers would "bid" competitively to draw on public funds.

The Regulatory Work Stream recommends that a package of such incentives and standalone funding be enacted into law to extend high speed broadband service to underserved areas, possibly as part of a major effort to restructure the rural health care sector in the United States as laid out in the payment chapter earlier in this report.

Net Neutrality

Further questions related to the issue of high speed broadband access arise over the implications of the Federal Communication Commission's recent repeal of the net neutrality rule adopted in 2015. Net neutrality is the principle that Internet service providers (ISP's) must treat all data on the Internet the same, and not discriminate; the provision had officially governed internet service since 2015, when broadband ISPs were classified as "common carriers" under federal communications law. In effect, the provision meant that ISPs could not allow some data users to access "fast lanes" for data transmission while blocking or otherwise discriminating against other material. As the "WIRED Guide to Net Neutrality" put it, companies like Comcast or Verizon shouldn't be able to block you from accessing a service like Skype [owned by Microsoft], or slow down Netflix or Hulu, in order to encourage you to keep your cable package [from Comcast] or buy a different video-streaming service [from Verizon or Amazon].[121]

In 2017, at the urging of FCC commissioner Ajit Pai, a Trump administration appointee, the commission voted to repeal the net neutrality rule; the repeal subsequently took full effect in spring 2018. The core question is what will happen in the marketplace next. Opponents of repeal predict that ISPs will now create different "lanes," requiring services that want to deliver data faster – or, for video, at higher levels of resolution—to pay higher rates that will ultimately be passed along to consumers. FCC commissioner Pai argues that the opposite will occur—that a less regulated market will create more choices for consumers and potentially lower data transmission charges—and that a separate agency, the Federal Trade Commission, will be able to "police internet service providers for anticompetitive acts and unfair or deceptive practices." [122]

A clear risk in a "Health Care Without Walls" future is that health data transmission over the internet might somehow be "throttled back" depending on the user who is transmitting it and that user's particular contract with the ISP. If Pai is correct, FTC oversight could provide some recourse against that happening. But until the post-net neutrality market fully evolves, and any new or different pricing structures or service agreements emerge, it is difficult to predict the future.

In the interim, a number of states have taken action to restore net neutrality within their borders. As of the publication of this report, legislators in 30 states have introduced more than 72 bills requiring internet service providers to ensure various net neutrality principles.[123] In 13 states and the District of Columbia, legislators introduced 23 resolutions primarily expressing opposition to the Federal Communications Commission's (FCC) repeal of net neutrality rules; urging the U.S. Congress to enact legislation reinstating and requiring the preservation of net neutrality; or stating the chamber's support of general net neutrality principles.

Governors in six states—Hawaii, New Jersey, New York, Montana, Rhode Island, and Vermont—have signed executive orders. Three states – Oregon, Vermont, and Washington, have enacted net neutrality legislation, and the California legislature adopted a net neutrality bill in late August 2018.

The Regulatory Work Stream recommended that this issue be watched carefully over the next several years to determine what the results are with respect to vital data and information transmission, including of health-related information, and the impact on costs for consumers, health care organizations dependent on data transmission, and others.

Summary Recommendations

The Regulatory Work Stream expressed the opinion that in general, new frameworks, models, and pathways are needed, or "islands of innovation" created, so that these new models of regulation can evolve and support the flourishing of more distributed health care systems. These regulatory models can and should be more focused on outcomes, and not so much on the conventional silos and "boxes"—such as those related to specific types of health care facilities—into which health care and attendant regulations have traditionally been packaged.

Key recommendations are the following:

1) Congress should enhance the authority of the Center for Medicare and Medicaid Innovation (CMMI) to experiment with new virtual care delivery models and engage states in these models as well. Although many aspects of innovative models deal with payment, as discussed in the previous chapter of this report, in some instances they could also require regulatory "safe harbors," such as under the Stark laws, that would permit health systems to provide useful technologies to providers and patients. One possible means of creating new delivery models would be building on the State Innovation Model grants in the Affordable Care Act to create a new version focused on distributed care models, particularly in rural areas of the nation, where a combination of new payment and regulatory approaches could be tested and evaluated.

2) A coalition of CMS, private payers, and health system leaders should develop sets of outcomes or objectives that new care delivery models should meet, and should take steps to ensure that these are applied nationwide (as with the Diabetes Prevention Program cited above). For example, one objective could be to deliver acute care that would traditionally be delivered in acute care settings such as hospitals, but in non-acute settings, such as homes, for comparable or superior quality and safety outcomes and 20 percent or even greater savings compared to conventional hospital stays (in effect,

Hospital at Home). Once again, certain regulatory safe harbors may need to be part and parcel of these delivery models.

3) The federal government should address certain regulatory obstacles to telehealth and telemedicine, such as the Drug Enforcement Administration regulations on prescribing of controlled substances described above. The DEA should move forward with its announced plan to adopt a single national telemedicine registration that would allow a prescriber to prescribe controlled substances via telemedicine anywhere in the nation. The federal government should also adopt limited safe harbors regarding the Anti-Kickback Statute and Stark Laws that would facilitate the provision of hardware, software, apps, and other low-cost technologies from health systems to physicians and patients, for the purposes of conducting more telemedicine or telehealth and distributed care. The federal government should also create incentives for states to act to remove barriers as well (e.g., prescribing rules, professional corporation rules, physical visit requirements) that militate against provision of telehealth and telemedicine.

4) As discussed in the Work Force Work Stream recommendations, model state statutes should be developed that expand the scope of practice for multiple types of health professionals, including advanced practice nurses, to make maximum and flexible use of the health care labor force. Once these model laws are developed, states should enact them.

5) The federal government should either develop a parallel system of national licensure of health care professionals, or it should create a quasi-public entity to enact new national licensure provisions and allow for voluntary licensure at this level for health care professionals. States could be incentivized, but not required, to adopt the new national or federal licensure standards as their own, or to cease state-based licensure and agree to let the national licensure system govern in their state.

6) Failing the approaches described above in recommendations (3) and (5), "innovation pacts" should be struck between and among states that have a common interest in creating greater fluidity of care—for example, in states that are parties to the movement of so-called "snowbirds," who may move between the north and south during the year in pursuit of good weather. For example, Florida and Michigan could agree to take a common approach on telehealth/telemedicine and various provider licensure issues to facilitate care flowing between providers and patients in those two states. These

compacts should take the form of the nursing licensure compact and allow a provider licensed in one state to automatically qualify for licensure in any other state that is a party to the pact or compact.

7) Again failing the approaches described above in recommendations (3), (5), and (6), above, the federal government should develop incentives for states to adopt interstate licensure compacts more rapidly, not just for health professionals but also for mail order pharmacies. More broadly, voluntary interstate regulatory compacts pertaining to a range of health care regulatory issues should be created, along the lines of what the FDA and states have done with respect to memorandums of understanding on certain regulatory issues.

8) Through training and certification programs and possibly licensure, states should expand the use of community health workers, as recommended in the Work Force chapter of this report. Such workers have a demonstrated track record of connecting well with individuals living in the community, and will be a vitally important source of support for them as they new care models evolve that employ greater use of technology.

9) To address health information privacy and security, Congress should address the complex array of federal, state, constitutional, statutory, and regulatory provisions that apply in the U.S., and do the following:

    - Create one health care federal privacy and security regulator and one overarching set of health and health care privacy and security regulations along the lines of the European Union's General Data Privacy Regulation (GDPR), as discussed above.

    - As it is not clear whether or not the creation of one health care privacy and security regulator would be possible in the US context, all companies producing devices or other entities that utilize or transmit health-related data and information should adopt a code of conduct around both health and health care data privacy and security and a self-regulatory obligation to meet standards and requirements of the FDA, the FTC, and other relevant federal and state regulatory agencies.

10) On device regulation by the FDA and the agency's pre-certification program, the FDA should continue to provide guidance as technology evolves on which devices it will regulate and which it will not. The pre-certification

program should be closely studied and expanded to other companies over time, particularly as those companies sign onto the industry-wide code of conduct on privacy and security as set forth above.

11) Federal and, to a large degree, state regulation of autonomous vehicles is virtually nonexistent at the moment, and there is particular need for clarity of regulation of medically equipped autonomous vehicles. Cooperative groups among government, industry, and representatives of the public should be empaneled to study what safety and other issues will arise and consider appropriate options for self-regulation or public sector regulation.

12) Access to high speed broadband is vital in today's society and economy, especially for the purposes of advancing public health and enabling a state-of-the art health care sector. It is unconscionable that much of the U.S. population lacks access to affordable high-speed broadband. Amid signs that a major national infrastructure investment plan may not be forthcoming, the Regulatory Work Stream recommends that Congress enact multiple approaches to extend high speed broadband service to underserved areas; these could include grants and loans to towns or rural cooperatives; tax credits to incentivize private companies to expand into underserved areas; and "reverse auctions," in which internet service providers would "bid" competitively to draw on public funds. The Regulatory Work Stream recommends that this package be considered as part of a major effort to restructure the rural health care sector in the United States as laid out in the payment chapter earlier in this report.

13) Amid uncertainties about whether the repeal of net neutrality provisions will increase or lower costs of data transmission over the internet, or advantage or disadvantage certain types of users, Congress should require the Federal Communications Commission and the Federal Trade Commission to jointly conduct annual studies of the effects of repeal on pricing and data transmission. If signs emerge that costs are rising excessively for certain types of users—whether they are groups of individuals, companies, or economic sectors—or that they are being "steered" into slower lanes of transmission in a way that results in deleterious effects, particularly on health care and public health, Congress should act to restore net neutrality as a national requirement.

Regulation and Health Care Without Walls: Chapter 3 in Brief

1. U.S. health care is a highly regulated enterprise at the federal, state, and even local level—the paramount reasons for which are the need to ensure a high level of health care quality and safety for consumers and patients, and protection against fraud. As a result, multiple regulatory issues at the federal, state, and local level will pertain to the movement of health care to more distributed settings, thanks to the vast array of regulations that govern the range of personnel who provide health care and who will be using technology; the places and settings in which technology-enabled care is provided; the technology-driven aspects of care that are provided; and technological equipment itself.

2. As health care evolves, well-intended regulations written for one era of health care pose uncertainties for technology-driven innovations that arise in another era. An example are hospital-at-home programs that are neither, strictly speaking, hospital care or home care, but may be subject to licensure requirements in states that apply differently to those activities. What's more, because much of health care now depends on exchanges of digital information, specific areas of regulation not unique to health care, but more generally applicable to information in general, now play an important role. Differences in regulation among countries also affect health care, such as new European Union information privacy and security standards.

3. A further complexity is that, in US health care, regulation is often very closely tied to payment. This particular duality—regulation tied to payment—creates special problems in the context of virtual care that is cutting across older care, reimbursement, and regulatory silos.

4. Taking into account the vision developed by the Technology Work Stream as to what the delivery of health care could look like in 2025, the Regulatory Work Stream of the Health Care Without Walls Initiative considered such topics as governmental approval of digital health products and devices; regulations governing privacy, security, and health information retention; and health professional licensure and scope of practice, among others. Its overall goal was to articulate a regulatory framework at the federal and state levels that would support evolution of a more distributed care system, and deliver the benefits of a more accessible, timely, convenient, and lower cost health care system while preserving or advancing quality and safety.

5. Recommendations of the Regulatory Work Stream extended across many different and evolving areas. In general, the work stream recommended, new frameworks, models, and pathways are needed, or "islands of innovation" created, so that these new models of regulation can evolve and support the flourishing of more distributed health care systems. These regulatory models can and should be more focused on outcomes for patients, and not so much on the conventional silos and "boxes"—such as those related to specific types of health care facilities—into which health care and attendant regulations have traditionally been packaged. An example would be enhancing the authority of the Center for Medicare and Medicaid Innovation (CMMI) to experiment with new virtual care delivery and payment models that could also require regulatory safe harbors, such as under the Stark Law, to permit health systems to provide useful technologies to providers.

6. The federal government should address certain regulatory obstacles to telemedicine, such as the Drug Enforcement Administration regulations on prescribing of controlled substances described above. The DEA should move forward with its announced plan to adopt a single national telemedicine registration that would allow a prescriber to prescribe controlled substances via telemedicine anywhere in the nation.

7. As discussed at greater length in the Work Force Work Stream recommendations, states should enact model statutes that expand the scope of practice for multiple types of health professionals, including advanced practice nurses, to make maximum and flexible use of the health care labor force in the delivery of more distributed care. Through certification programs and possibly licensure, states should expand use of community health workers, as recommended in the Work Force chapter of this report. The federal government should either develop a parallel system of national licensure of health care professionals, or create a quasi-public entity that to enact new national licensure provisions, to allow for voluntary licensure at this level for health care professionals. States could be incentivized, but not required, to adopt the new national or federal licensure standards as their own, or to cease state-based licensure and agree to let the national licensure system govern in their state. Failing that approach, "innovation pacts" should be struck between and among states that have a common interest in creating greater fluidity of care—for example, in states that are parties to the movement of so-called "snowbirds," who may move between the north and south during the year in pursuit of good weather.

8. To address health information privacy and security, Congress should address the complex array of federal, state, constitutional, statutory, and regulatory provisions that apply in the U.S., and do the following:

   - Create one health care federal privacy and security regulator and one overarching set of health and health care privacy and security regulations along the lines of the European Union's General Data Privacy Regulation (GDPR), as discussed above.

   - If the creation of one health care privacy and security regulator is impossible in the U.S. context, all companies producing devices or other entities that utilize or transmit health-related data and information should adopt a code of conduct around both health and health care data privacy and security and a self-regulatory obligation to meet standards and requirements of the FDA, the FTC, and other relevant federal and state regulatory agencies.

9. Autonomous cars may eventually play a major role in the delivery of health care, but federal and, to a large degree, state regulation of them is virtually nonexistent at the moment. Cooperative groups among government, industry, and representatives of the public should be empaneled to study what safety and other issues will arise and consider appropriate options for self-regulation or public sector regulation.

10. On device regulation by the FDA and the agency's pre-certification program, the FDA should continue to provide guidance as technology evolves on which devices it will regulate and which it will not. The pre-certification program should be closely studied and expanded to other companies over time, particularly as those companies sign onto the industry-wide code of conduct on privacy and security as set forth above.

11. Access to high speed broadband is vital in today's society and economy, especially for the purposes of advancing public health and enabling a state-of-the art health care sector. It is unconscionable that much of the U.S. population lacks access to affordable high-speed broadband. Amid signs that a major national infrastructure investment plan is unlikely to be forthcoming in the short term, Congress should enact multiple approaches to extend high speed broadband service to underserved areas; these could include grants and loans to towns or rural cooperatives; tax credits to incentivize private companies to expand into underserved areas; and "reverse auctions," in

which internet service providers would "bid" competitively to draw on public funds.

12. Amid uncertainties about whether the repeal of net neutrality provisions will increase or lower costs of data transmission over the internet, or advantage or disadvantage certain types of users, Congress should require the Federal Communications Commission and the Federal Trade Commission to jointly conduct annual studies of the effects of repeal on pricing and data transmission, including comparisons among states that have or have not acted to preserve net neutrality. If signs emerge that costs are rising excessively for certain types of users—whether they are groups of individuals, companies, or economic sectors—or that they are being "steered" into slower lanes of transmission in a way that results in deleterious effects, particularly on health care and public health, Congress should act to restore net neutrality as a national requirement.

♦ ♦ ♦

End Notes, Chapter 3

[89] See https://www.cms.gov/Medicare/Provider-Enrollment-and-Certification/SurveyCertificationGenInfo/Downloads/Survey-and-Cert-Letter-18-10.pdf.

[90] See https://figure1.com; also https://en.wikipedia.org/wiki/Figure_1.

[91] "State Telehealth Laws and Reimbursement Policies," Center for Connected Health Policy, The National Telehealth Policy Resource Center (April 2017):5, http://www.cchpca.org/sites/default/files/resources/50%20STATE%20PDF%20FILE%20APRIL%202017%20FINAL%20PASSWORD%20PROTECT.pdf.

[92] "Putting Patients First: Spurring Health Care Innovation through Regulatory Modernization," New York State Department of Health Regulatory Modernization Initiative, February 2018, https://www.health.ny.gov/regulations/regulatory_modernization_initiative/docs/regulatory_modernization_initiative_report_2017.pdf.

[93] Diabetes Prevention Program (DPP) Research Group, "The Diabetes Prevention Program (DPP): description of lifestyle intervention," *Diabetes Care* 25, no. 12 (2002): 2165-2171.

[94] Nathaniel Lacktman, "Telemedicine Prescribing and Controlled Substances Laws," Health Care Law Today, April 3, 2017, https://www.healthcarelawtoday.com/2017/04/03/telemedicine-prescribing-and-controlled-substances-laws/.

[95] U.S. Department of Justice, Drug Enforcement Administration, Diversion Control Division, "Title 21 United State Code Controlled Substances Act", *Chapter 13 - Drug Abuse Prevention and Control, Subchapter 1 - Control and Enforcement*, 2016, https://www.deadiversion.usdoj.gov/21cfr/21usc/index.html.

[96] "Digital health innovation action plan," Center for Devices & Radiological Health, U.S. Food and Drug Administration (2017): 2, https://www.fda.gov/downloads/MedicalDevices/DigitalHealth/UCM568735.pdf.

[97] Evan Sweeney, "After a 6-year Wait, FDA's Clinical Decision Support Guidelines get a Mixed Reaction," Fierce Healthcare December 7, 2017, https://www.fiercehealthcare.com/regulatory/fda-clinical-decision-support-bradley-merrill-thompson-bethany-hills-ai-21st-century.

[98] Ibid.

[99] Vincent Liu, Mark A. Musen, and Timothy Chou, "Data Breaches of Protected Health Information in the United States," *JAMA* 313, no.14(April 14, 2015):1471-1473, DOI: 10.1001/jama.2015.2252.

[100] Liz Sly et al., "U.S. Military Reviewing its Rules after Fitness Trackers Exposed Sensitive Data," The Washington Post, January 29, 2018, https://www.washingtonpost.com/world/the-us-military-reviews-its-rules-as-new-details-of-us-soldiers-and-bases-emerge/2018/01/29/6310d518-050f-11e8-aa61-f3391373867e_story.html?utm_term=.69723bdb2e66.

[101] Hamza Shaban, "An Amazon Echo recorded a family's conversation, then sent it to a random person in their contacts, reports says," The Washington Post, May 24, 2018, https://www.washingtonpost.com/news/the-switch/wp/2018/05/24/an-amazon-echo-recorded-a-familys-conversation-then-sent-it-to-a-random-person-in-their-contacts-report-says/?utm_term=.b9fd97fbd9eb.

[102] Janine Hiller et al., "Privacy and Security in the Implementation of Health Information Technology (Electronic Health Records): U.S. and EU compared," *Boston University Journal of Science and Technology* (2011): 1, https://www.bu.edu/jostl/files/2015/02/Hiller_Web_171.pdf.

[103] US Department of Health and Human Services, Office for Civil Rights, the Office of the National Coordinator for Health Information Technology, "Permitted Uses and Disclosures: Exchange for Treatment," *45 Code of Federal Regulations* 164.506(c)(2), (January 2016), https://www.healthit.gov/sites/default/files/exchange_treatment.pdf.

[104] See https://en.wikipedia.org/wiki/FTC_fair_information_practice.

[105] Elin B. Begley et al., "Personally Identifiable Information in State Laws: Use, Release, and Collaboration at Health Departments," *American Journal of Public Health* 107, no.8(August 2017):1272-1276, DOI: 10.2105/AJPH.2017.303862.

[106] See https://leginfo.legislature.ca.gov/faces/billTextClient.xhtml?bill_id=201720180AB375.

[107] "Federal Trade Commission Spring Privacy Series: Consumer Generated and Controlled Health Data," May 7, 2014, https://www.ftc.gov/system/files/documents/public_events/195411/2014_05_07_consumer-generated-controlled-health-data-final-transcript.pdf.

[108] "Preparing for the Future of Artificial Intelligence," Executive Office of the President, National Science and Technology Council October 2016, https://obamawhitehouse.archives.gov/sites/default/files/whitehouse_files/microsites/ostp/NSTC/preparing_for_the_future_of_ai.pdf.

[109] "Clinical and Patient Decision Support Software," US Food and Drug Administration, (December 2017),

https://www.fda.gov/downloads/MedicalDevices/DeviceRegulationandGuidance/GuidanceDocuments/UCM587819.pdf.

[110] Dolores Derrington, "Artificial Intelligence for Health and Health Care," The Mitre Corporation, (December 2017), https://www.healthit.gov/sites/default/files/jsr-17-task-002_aiforhealthandhealthcare12122017.pdf.

[111] Software as a Medical Device Working Group, "Software as a Medical Device: Clinical Evaluation," *International Medical Device Regulators Forum* (August 2016), http://www.imdrf.org/docs/imdrf/final/consultations/imdrf-cons-samd-ce.pdf.

[112] See http://cdscoalition.org/wp-content/uploads/2017/08/CDS-3060-Guidelines-Final-2.pdf.

[113] Nicholas Diakopoulos and Sorelle Friedler, "How to Hold Algorithms Accountable," MIT Technology Review, November 17, 2016, https://www.technologyreview.com/s/602933/how-to-hold-algorithms-accountable/.

[114] Colin Lecher, "What Happens When An Algorithm Cuts Your Health Care," The Verge, March 21, 2018, https://www.theverge.com/2018/3/21/17144260/healthcare-medicaid-algorithm-arkansas-cerebral-palsy.

[115] Ibid.

[116] "AMA Passes First Policy Recommendations on Augmented Intelligence," AMA, June 14, 2018, https://www.ama-assn.org/ama-passes-first-policy-recommendations-augmented-intelligence.

[117] See http://www.oecd.org/sti/broadband/broadband-statistics/.

[118] Lennard Kruger et al., "Broadband Internet Access and the Digital Divide: Federal Assistance Programs," Congressional Research Service, December 2016, https://fas.org/sgp/crs/misc/RL30719.pdf.

[119] Federal Communications Commission, "FCC-NCI Broadband Cancer Collaboration," Connect 2 Health FCC, November 2017, https://www.fcc.gov/health/cancer.

[120] See https://docs.fcc.gov/public/attachments/DOC-352655A1.pdf.

[121] Klint Finley, "The Wired Guide to Net Neutrality," Wired, May 9, 2018, https://www.wired.com/story/guide-net-neutrality/.

[122] Ajit Pai, "FCC chairman:Our job is to protect a free and open internet," CNET, June 10, 2018, https://www.cnet.com/news/fcc-chairman-our-job-is-to-protect-a-free-and-open-internet/.

[123] See "Net Neutrality Legislation in States," National Conference of State Legislatures, at http://www.ncsl.org/research/telecommunications-and-information-technology/net-neutrality-legislation-in-states.aspx.

SCENARIO 6: A WOMAN RECOVERING FROM BREAST CANCER

STEPHANIE IS A 62-year-old woman who recently completed treatment with radiation and chemotherapy for stage 2 breast cancer. She is divorced, and lives in a suburban area of a booming Southeastern city. College educated, and with what was once a middle-class income, she was recently laid off and is currently on COBRA. She is mildly depressed but hopes to recover sufficiently to find a new job with health coverage. She has a smart phone, and an old computer and printer, and is computer-savvy enough to be using the internet to search for a job and participate in online cancer patient support groups.

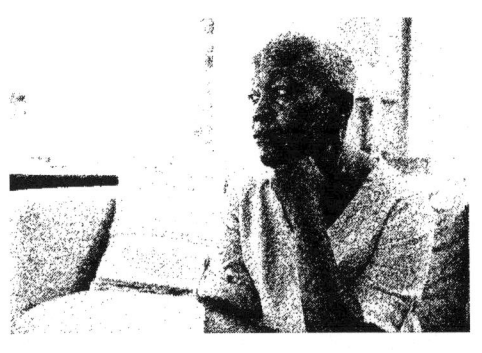

More than 252,000 women like Stephanie, and nearly 2,500 men, are diagnosed with breast cancer each year in the United States. Breast cancer is the most commonly diagnosed cancer in women and the second leading cause of cancer death in women. There has been a gradual reduction in female breast cancer incidence rates among women aged 50 and older, and death rates from breast cancer have been declining since about 1990, in part due to better screening, early detection, and improvements in treatment, including targeted therapies.

Fortunately, Stephanie's community oncology practice participated in a local oncology medical home model. In an atypical collaboration, Stephanie's care coordinator from the medical home, and a case manager with Stephanie's health plan, have devised a list of optimal care goals for Stephanie. Job one is to maintain and assist in Stephanie's recovery from breast cancer, including treating her depression and enabling her to return to work. Stephanie will also need regular mammograms and other checkups. Her immune system will remain somewhat compromised for a while, because of the chemotherapy, so Stephanie's clinical care team must be on close watch for any infections.

As Stephanie's care is handed off from the oncology medical home, to a patient-centered, primary care medical home, more coordination ensues. Stephanie's health plan pays for telehealth consultations with both Stephanie's oncologist and her primary care provider. Stephanie also has regular Skype visits with a psychiatric social worker to help her deal with her depression, and a wellness expert who has instructed her on stress reduction techniques. A lifestyle coach has helped her get back into a regular exercise routine. As Stephanie's depression lifts, she also consults with a job coach, to which she was also referred by her health plan, for assistance in her job search.

A tip from a nurse practitioner on her care team has also proved invaluable. Stephanie learned about an app that provides information about clinical trials in which former breast cancer patients can enroll, to study the effects of being on certain medications following breast cancer. Stephanie completes several forms online, and is ultimately matched to a clinical trial. This one is to be conducted almost entirely virtually: Patients will only need to participate in their standard follow-up, post-cancer care; results of tests will be reported to the clinical trial coordinator; and Stephanie will report in regularly on any symptoms via an app.

Participating in the trial boosts Stephanie's sense that something good might come of her cancer, and that she'll be able to contribute to medical knowledge that will help other breast cancer sufferers in the future. Stephanie thinks to herself: Life is looking up.

◆ ◆ ◆

CHAPTER 4:
THE WORK FORCE TO SUPPORT HEALTH CARE WITHOUT WALLS

As previous chapters in this report have laid out, NEHI's vision for health care in 2025 is that health care will increasingly be accessed and delivered "without walls." Patients will receive more care than they do now in their homes, schools, and other community-based venues and "distributed" settings out of conventional health care settings, such as hospitals and physicians' offices; vast amounts of data will be turned into actionable information to assist clinical decision-making; care will be delivered far more often than at present by multidisciplinary teams of providers, whose clinical competencies will be accompanied by new skill sets that facilitate application of technology and informatics in routine patient care; and these multidisciplinary teams will also address the social and economic determinants of health that often drive illness and care needs. All of these changes will have a profound impact on the health care work force.

Although it is impossible to predict fully what the future health care work force will look like, or how it will function, several imperatives will loom large. New capabilities and practices will have to be created to provide excellent health care in more distributed settings; more types of workers, such as community health workers, may be needed, and the tasks performed by current types of workers, in terms of what they do and how they do it, will change. At the same time, because labor represents such a large cost component of health care, keeping that care affordable will demand increased productivity of labor, not simply having more bodies providing it. Advancing technology may provide opportunities both to supplant some types of labor, as well as to augment the decision-making skills of health professionals to such a degree that "task shifting" of labor from higher-skilled to less-skilled workers may also become a reality.

Examples of anticipated changes that will affect how health care workers do their jobs and perform tasks include the following:

- Patients will travel to physician offices and other institutional settings less frequently to receive care as they interact more with providers directly from their homes, schools, work sites, and other community and "distributed" settings.

- Virtual health care platforms will enable health professionals to deliver needed services from anywhere, a change that will at least somewhat reduce the role of hospitals and doctors' offices as the physical locations in which care is provided.

- Data gathered both inside and outside conventional clinical settings—from electronic health records, to patients' own sensor-equipped smart watches, for example—will be combined and analyzed to provide health care teams with a more complete picture of a patient's physical and social circumstances, thereby facilitating more informed decisions about what services and supports are needed.

- Providers will respond to both urgent and routine care needs and triage patients through new technology-enabled systems, and they will increasingly send appropriate health professionals and aides to the home if, and when, they are needed.

- New partnerships among health systems, pharmacies, schools, employers, community health centers, and others, will deliver targeted care where it is needed by marshalling local resources to provide care in new ways.

- Ongoing and strategic reallocation of labor will result from thoughtful analysis of what kinds of skills and training are needed throughout the health care labor force, how to make determinations based on this analysis, and implementing appropriate changes in the proportions of physicians, nurses, and other health professionals.

- It will be increasingly important to have all health professionals, and particularly non-physician health care professionals, trained, certified, and empowered to practice at the top of their licenses.

- Improved training and education, as well as the ability for health care professionals to work at the top of their licenses, will result in task-shifting—the "process whereby specific tasks are moved, where appropriate, to health workers with shorter training and fewer qualifications."[124]

- There will be a greatly expanded role for community pharmacists, community health workers, and other types of workers who will create a new "front line" in health care closer to individuals in their homes and communities. Such workers will establish and maintain links between patients and other care team members, and facilitate patients' access to community-based resources.

- The roles of almost all types of health care professionals are likely to change substantially, and it will be critical to have the health care work force be as flexible and adaptable as possible. Much of the health care work force is arguably already underutilized in many parts of the country; with new avenues of care opening up through information and technology, new opportunities exist to use this work force much more efficiently and effectively.

To achieve this vision for 2025, the health care work force must evolve in response to dramatic trends that are already under way. These trends include the rapid evolution of health-related information technology, including information that will enhance delivery of precision medicine; demographic trends that yield increasing numbers of older, medically complex patients; broader recognition of how social and environmental factors impact health; and profound shifts in consumer expectations and preferences concerning how and where they want to receive health care supports and services. To meet these challenges, America's health care work force needs to update its collective skill set, a far-reaching goal that will not be achieved quickly or easily. Attaining this goal will require the following interventions:

- **Education and training** infrastructure in which faculty in degree-granting programs have the knowledge and skills to provide instruction on health informatics, virtual health care, team-based care, and working in collaboration with community-based organizations.

- **Continuing education** for existing health care professionals that allows them to obtain the necessary skills to deliver more virtual, team-based care, and to function effectively in a rapidly-changing health care environment.

- **Expanded online education** that allow aspiring health professionals—especially low-income students and those in rural areas—to access high-quality, relevant, education that provides appropriate preparation for entry into the work force of the future.

- **Defining and filling new types of jobs** that will be needed under a more distributed, technology-driven health care system.

- **Addressing state licensure requirements and scope-of-practice laws** that militate against effective use of all levels of providers in practicing virtual care.

None of these essential elements for future development of the health care work force is currently in place to an adequate degree. As a result, health care professionals—those who are currently in practice as well as those who are enrolled in or aspire to enter school or other certificate programs—may not be fully prepared to meet the challenges that lie ahead.

Unless these shortcomings are addressed, they will prevent Americans from fully benefiting from the many ways that technology and a more distributed health care system can promote health and well-being. Beyond the favorable impact on public health of a re-imagined health care work force, there are additional public policy considerations: Health systems and payers will ultimately incur unnecessary costs that can be avoided if the health care work force is prepared to fully employ technology and new ways of delivering care.

The Scope of Work for the "Health Care Without Walls" Work Force Work Stream

Toward the goals of improving individual and population health, strengthening communities, increasing quality of health care, and controlling costs, the Work Force Work Stream of the Health Care Without Walls initiative was charged with the following tasks:

1. Taking into account the vision developed by the Technology Work Stream (see Chapter 2) as to what the delivery of health care could look like in 2025, articulate a vision for a qualified work force capable of meeting the health and health care needs of Americans at that time.

2. Articulate a vision of a work force that advances the *health* of Americans, not just the care.

3. Determine what types of education and training will prepare the future work force to provide safe, efficacious, efficient, accessible, cost-effective, and culturally appropriate care in distributed settings.

4. Identify a process and methodology for determining appropriate types and numbers of competent health workers, given uncertainties about how technology may be implemented and used.

5. Identify any critical research gaps about the health care work force that must be filled as we move to a system of Health Care Without Walls. How will an evidence base for delivery of virtual care be developed; by whom; and according to what timetable?

6. Draft a set of recommendations for changes in public policy and within health care organizations, payers, and others, to support the 2025 work force vision.

The Value of a Technology-Enabled Health Care Work Force

To describe accurately the impact of technology on the future health care work force, it is first necessary to define what the term "technology" means in the context of this report. As noted in the Technology chapter of this report, when Health Care Without Walls refers to "technologies," it includes information technologies that gather and/or transmit data and information, or that use digital information in novel ways.

Technology is therefore considered in the broadest sense, to include items that are conventionally deemed technology—such as robotics or smart devices—as well as the entire digital universe of artificial or augmented intelligence, cognitive computing, and information analytics. Thus, a more comprehensive list of technologies includes the following:

- Telehealth and telemedicine

- Software, such as SaMD (software with a medical purpose)

- Data and information exchange

- Clinical decision support (CDS) systems

- Artificial or augmented intelligence, cognitive computing, and machine learning

- Internet-enabled health devices and the Internet of Things

- Mobile medical applications; medical device data systems, used for the electronic transfer, storage, display, or conversion of medical device data; medical image storage devices, used to store or retrieve medical images electronically; and medical image communications devices, used to transfer medical image data electronically between medical devices

- "Low-risk" general wellness products, such as apps

- Lab tests, such as self-administered tests, and other technologies involved with laboratory work flow

- Autonomous cars

- Robots and robotics

- Drones

Most Americans who engage with today's health care system can point to numerous technological changes that have occurred in recent years. Patient information is often collected and stored in electronic health records (EHRs); growing numbers of patients get their prescription medications through electronic prescribing (e-prescribing); and patients can often access their health information, request prescription refills, and schedule appointments using web-based portals.

Although these technological advances have provided meaningful benefits to patients, they have also required health care professionals to interact with data, with patients, and with one another in new ways. In addition, they have required health care professionals and other health care workers to learn new, non-clinical skills that are linked to a wide variety of health-related technologies. Yet adapting to some of these technologies, such as EHRs, has proven difficult for many providers for multiple reasons, ranging from the lack of usability of some technologies, to resistance to changing work habits or disruptions to existing patterns of clinical work flow.[125] The health care work force's inability to fully optimize the use of technologies such as EHRs raises obvious concerns about how these diverse groups of workers will harness other technologies to address the health and clinical care challenges that lie ahead.

As stakeholders—particularly professional societies and institutions of health professions education and training—begin to address the practical challenges that will stem from ensuring that their constituencies are prepared for the changes that lie ahead, these organizations need to think through how new technologies, automation, augmented intelligence and other technological advances will change the tasks in which existing workers routinely engage.

As discussed further below, the application of artificial intelligence to radiology has already highlighted the fact that many scans can be more accurately "read" by machines than by humans. The application of AI in radiology is only one example of a larger trend characterized by increased use of, and reliance on AI for clinical decision support (CDS). As these CDS systems continue to evolve, there will be parallel changes in how health care workers interact with these systems in delivering care. It is likely that AI-driven changes will be most noticeable for routine tasks in which there is limited patient-to-patient variability, or tasks for which decision-making can be enhanced by new information that can be incorporated by AI into care planning.

For example, by incorporating home-based sensor data that provides insight on patients' risk of falling, AI could be used to enhance decision support for medication management, especially for older adults. AI and predictive analytics could be also used to help care teams better predict a patient's health trajectory after surgery so that the patient and their family can plan in advance for needed services and supports.

Increased use of AI comes with the need to acknowledge that in many cases, AI-driven decision-making can facilitate delivery of certain types of routine care by health care workers who are at a lower level than those who currently deliver these services. As a result, the ongoing incorporation of AI into CDS will not only require a critical evaluation of health care workers' education, training, and licensure, but it will also fuel a larger discussion about which types of workers can and should be engaged in specific tasks, as well as when, and how they engage in these tasks (see discussion of task shifting, pp, 191-193).

As a result of all of these changes and concerns, the Health Care Without Walls has advanced a vision of health care for America in 2025 that will be characterized by a health care work force that optimizes technology to deliver health care—*both health and care*—in a manner that is more distributed, efficient, and patient-centered than it is today. This vision relies heavily on using all proven health and information technologies that are available, and creating mechanisms to incorporate new technologies in the future.

To achieve this vision, the health care work force must be educated and trained in the new and emerging health and information technologies that will characterize health care delivery in the United States in the future. Health care professionals also must be able to access and benefit from continuing education that is rich in technology and informatics. They must be able to work at the top of their licenses and certifications, and they must no longer be hindered from delivering needed care by outdated regulations that are based on older models of care delivery; unrealistic attitudes about the virtues of in-person care versus virtual care; clinging to geographic boundaries; or desires to restrict competition. Many of these factors are outmoded and have little or no practical relevance in an increasingly connected world.

The recommendations offered at the end of this chapter have the potential to position America's health care work force, so it can optimize current and future health technology for the benefit of all Americans. If implemented, these recommendations would result in far-reaching changes that offer benefits to diverse stakeholders, highlighting the value of a technology-enabled and data-driven health care work force. Together with other needed changes, as spelled out in the reports of the other work streams involved in this project, these changes in the health care work force could accomplish the following:

- **Increase access to care**

    A health care work force that fully utilized technology could markedly increase access to care. People who live in rural areas could receive preventive and follow-up care with telemedicine or telehealth visits. Clinicians could bring primary care to low-income communities with technology-enabled mobile clinics. Rather than being admitted to nursing homes, older adults could receive appropriate, in-home care from multidisciplinary teams of clinicians and social services providers coordinated by technology platforms that respond in real time to patients' evolving needs. Indeed, models of such care already exist in multiple sites around the country (see Technology chapter pp. 31 to 72).

- **Rationalize the distribution of labor in the health care market**

Labor is the single biggest source of cost in the health care system, constituting about a half of average hospital costs, for example. At the same time, licensure, credentialing, and other well-intentioned features of regulation that are designed to guarantee a certain level of skills can also lock workers into a rigid set of tasks that hinders development of a labor pool with the capacity to respond to changing short- and long-term needs. These limitations are compounded by a lack of regulatory harmonization across states that limits flexibility even more. Furthermore, there is no mechanism to purposefully engage in an ongoing examination aimed at ensuring that health care labor is allocated appropriately across the entirety of the health care system.

Reducing health care costs, or holding them to a reasonable rate of growth, clearly must involve extracting costs from labor, ideally by increasing the productivity of labor in the system. To accomplish this goal, the concepts of "jobs" and "tasks" must be distinguished from one another. For example, in the current health care system, it may fall to a prescribing clinician to counsel a patient on the importance of adhering to a medication regimen, but that is a task that need not necessarily go hand-in-hand with the "job" of being a physician or nurse practitioner, and might be more efficiently executed by someone else, such as a pharmacist. Especially in the environment of rapidly changing technology, this distinction between jobs and tasks must be an ongoing process that leads to the distribution of labor throughout the health care system to those who can carry out processes most efficiently, and cost effectively.

Although it is difficult to predict how systematic separation of jobs and tasks, and reassignment of tasks to those who can carry them out most cost effectively, would play out for specific segments of the health care work force, it is likely that some tasks would be shifted from certain workers to others, and that certain jobs and tasks would also be displaced outright by technology. The Work Force Work Stream agreed that the fundamental need for physicians, nurses, pharmacists, and many other categories of health workers will not disappear in the future, but the group also believed that the tasks that these groups perform will shift considerably.

- **Making Fuller and More Effective Use of the Existing Provider Base**

It is well understood that the nation suffers from a maldistribution of many types of health care workers, who, like the rest of the population, tend to cluster in urban centers. The result is that there are thousands of health professional shortage areas (HPSAs), as well as medically underserved areas and populations (MUAs and MUPs), across the country. Specialists are among those most highly concentrated in urban areas, which means that access to some of the most sophisticated medical knowledge in the country is not always broadly available elsewhere. This maldistribution is compounded by the fact that non-physician segments of the health care work force are not fully utilized in their ability to deliver services, often because state laws restrict these providers from working at the top of their licenses, or because limitations on reimbursement affect their ability to provide and be paid for provision of services.

For example, advanced practice nurses can practice full care in just 22 states and the District of Columbia.[126] The resulting supply of unused potential in America's corps of advanced practice nurses, as well as in other aspects of the existing health care provider base, could be harnessed to deliver much needed primary care and support services. Similarly, although pharmacists have expanded their practice to provide a broad array of services such as medication management and administering immunizations, and can enter collaborative practice agreements with a physician or another prescriber in 47 states and the District of Columbia, they have limited ability to be reimbursed directly by Medicare and other payers for service that are provided within their scope of practice.[127]

If such scope-of-practice and reimbursement issues could be dealt with, health technology could enhance the impact of these and other workers even further by allowing them to deliver care virtually, in technology-enabled mobile clinics, or using other strategies that optimize health professionals' education and training for the benefit of those who need care.

- **Maximize support of family caregivers**

    Although this report places considerable emphasis on how technology will affect the professional health care work force in the future, the Work Force Work Stream also stressed the importance of recognizing the role of family and other informal caregivers, and optimizing their work via technology as well. The economic value of the health care services that are provided by informal caregivers—most often the family, friends, or neighbors of the patient—is measured in the hundreds of billions of dollars; if this assistance were not provided free by friends, families, and others, these costs would otherwise be borne by other parts of the health care system.

    Thus, the ability of informal caregivers to fully realize all the benefits that technology can offer helps shield the formal health care system from costs that are absorbed by informal support. Technology also allows informal caregivers to more easily access formal care when it is needed, thereby helping informal care recipients remain in the place they call home. Moreover, these technologies help maintain the health and well-being of the caregiver, allowing them to remain in their caregiving role as long as possible. Those in need of care are also enabled to stay in their own homes and communities, where most would prefer to be.

- **Fully support patient self-care**

    Although access to appropriate preventive and other formal health care services is a cornerstone of good health and recovery from illness, patients also have a central role in optimizing their own health, and in positioning themselves to recover from illness. As noted in the Technology chapter of this report, technology already plays a large role in how patients engage in these self-care efforts. Apps that help patients monitor their caloric intake and exercise are widely used, as are devices such as continuous positive airway pressure (CPAP) machines and glucose meters and pumps. In the future, these and other new technologies will play a larger role not only in how patients care for themselves, but also in how care teams access new kinds of data from these self-care technologies, and how this information is incorporated into care planning. The expansion of technology-enabled self-care strategies will therefore not only reinforce patients' roles in their own health maintenance, they will also provide new, and rich sources of data that can be incorporated into health records in ways that optimize care planning and clinical decision support.

- **Maximize quality of care**

    A health care work force with greater access to technology and improved training in informatics would be able to better track and interpret health information; deliver more "precision" medicine calibrated to an individual's specific genetics or other personalized information; improve coordination of care; reduce medical errors; and employ decision support at the point of care. Primary care providers in rural areas would be able to access specialty consults whenever they were needed. Home-based sensors or other digital devices could gather relevant information from patients and direct it to their care providers for analysis and incorporation into medical decision-making. In 2025, a re-imagined health care work force would fully employ these and other health care technologies to improve the overall quality of care by linking all members of the care team, including providers of social services and supports.

- **Deliver needed services at the appropriate time and in the most suitable place**

    Technology provides an important opportunity to challenge traditional notions concerning how quickly health professionals can deliver needed care, as well as the most "appropriate" settings in which providers can and should deliver services. Historically, many patients have had to endure long wait times to receive care, and this care was delivered mostly in such institutional settings as hospitals, physician offices, and nursing homes. Patients often need to leave work to access care – producing a productivity loss for the economy—or to travel long distances for care, imposing both costs and inconvenience on them. Technology-driven care—particularly virtual health care—means that providers can deliver needed care faster, and without the constraints of having to be physically located in a specific site. These advances allow providers to deliver services in the home or workplace, and in novel community settings such as churches and community centers. In many cases, these delivery strategies are not only received more favorably by patients, they are also less expensive and inconvenient.

- **Address upstream drivers of poor health**

    As noted in previous chapters of this report, there is ample evidence that a host of non-physiologic and non-behavioral factors (e.g. economic stability, neighborhood and physical environment, food access, education, etc.) have a direct and profound impact on human health.[128] Despite their impact on health, these factors are too rarely considered—much less addressed—in care planning. In 2025, Health Care Without Walls envisions an integrated, team-based, and technology-driven service delivery environment that acknowledges the social and economic determinants of health, and addresses them in parallel with traditional physiologic and behavioral risk factors. A re-imagined health care work force with new skills and knowledge concerning the intersection of technology, informatics, and social and economic risk factors would fully integrate community health workers, social workers, and new types of workers such as "health and wellness technology liaisons" (see further discussion below) to address upstream drivers of health as part of holistic, coordinated care planning.

- **Offer high-quality, lower-cost strategies that address challenging demographic trends**

    Well-known demographic trends, such as the aging of the U.S. population, could be effectively addressed by a health care work force that has fully employed technology to deliver services in the setting where these services are needed. Long-term care supports and services that are appropriately delivered in the home to growing numbers of frail seniors are more cost-effective than institutional care, which is often covered by public payers like Medicaid; indeed, such home and community-based services now constitute the largest share of overall Medicaid spending on long-term services and supports (in 2014, 53 percent, or $80.6 billion, of all Medicaid long term care spending was on home & community-based services)[129].

    Similarly, using technology and a refashioned health care work force to facilitate care delivery to rural communities—which are often poor and medically underserved—as well as service delivery to urban neighborhoods that are marginalized from the health care system, also have the potential to improve health and reduce downstream costs for public payers.

- **Increase the rewarding aspects of working in the health care sector**

    The current health care work force experiences a variety of frustrations that reduce job satisfaction and that ultimately may affect the supply of workers that is available to meet existing needs. These frustrations include the impact on clinical care of insufficient access to critical patient information at the point of care; discomfort with being forced to use technologies in real-world practice for which they have insufficient training; ongoing difficulties in addressing the health-related consequences of "upstream" social and environmental factors that can undermine patients' health; and a sense among some sectors of the health care work force that they are not practicing at their full potential.

Each of these frustrations could be addressed in a more distributed, coordinated, and technology-enabled health system in which education and training meet actual work place demands, and where providers deliver care at the top of their licenses using delivery models that take advantage of innovative technologies and that also address the complex interplay of social, economic, and physiologic factors on patients' health and care. Ultimately, a reduction in factors that diminish job satisfaction among health care workers will help ensure a vibrant work force well into the future.

Vision of a Health Care Work Force that Advances both Health and Care

In responding to Work Force Work Stream Goals #1 and 2, the group first articulated an overarching vision of a health care work force that can meet Americans' health and care needs in a manner consistent with the Health Care Without Walls 2025 vision. After articulating its overarching health care work force vision for 2025, the Work Force Work Stream identified a set of core principles that must be embodied by the 2025 health care work force if this vision is to be achieved.

> **Overarching vision of a health care work force capable of meeting
> the health and care needs of Americans in 2025:**
>
> **Health Care Without Walls envisions a health care work force that is educated and trained to optimize technology and health informatics, and that works at the top of license to deliver high-quality, team-based, and coordinated health care in settings that are clinically appropriate and impose the fewest restrictions and costs on patients and their families.**

To achieve this overarching vision, the 2025 health care work force must reflect the following core principles:

- Health care should be based on a fundamental platform of excellent primary care, and on integrating traditional clinical service streams with community-based social service providers to respond to the needs of the "whole person."

- Health care workers should be educated and trained about, and able to respond to, the social and economic determinants of health as a routine aspect of overall care planning.

- Health care workers should receive education and training that enable them to work effectively in technology-rich, data-driven, multidisciplinary teams whose efforts are coordinated and responsive to patients' evolving needs.

- Health care workers should be trained to deliver care at the top of their licenses, thereby enabling physicians to focus on care delivery and other issues that can best be handled by professionals with this level of education and training, and reserving other tasks to be carried out by many other types of health care workers.

- Health care workers should be organized into culturally competent teams that deliver appropriate combinations of in-person and virtual services. They should provide care in the least restrictive environment that is able to support meeting the goals of treatment.

To facilitate the development of recommendations for policy makers and other stakeholders, the Work Force Work Stream identified a seven-part framework of specific changes that will allow the health care work force to move toward achieving the Health Care Without Walls vision for 2025. The elements of this framework are (1) new models of care; (2) new roles and expanded scope of practice for existing health care workers; (3) the potential for task-shifting among existing types of workers; (4) the potential for disappearance of certain jobs and tasks; (5) the development of new types of health care workers; (6) recognizing the potential for changing employer-employee relationships broadly in the economy, and in health care in particular; and (7) updated education and training that will be necessary to address all of these considerations.

The discussion below elaborates on these elements and the implications for the health care work force.

1. **New Models of Care**

In 2025, advances in health information and technology will allow Americans unprecedented access to health care and supportive services, and this access will occur through models of care delivery that could not have been imagined just a decade ago. These new care models will employ many aspects of information and technology, including features that will allow these systems to be responsive to future clinical and technological innovation. It is likely that these models will share common elements that reflect the growing role of technology in care delivery.

These new approaches will influence how and where health care workers perform their roles; how different groups of health care workers collaborate with one another; and how these workers interact with community-based and other non-traditional organizations that should play larger roles in the future health care landscape. The following changes are likely to take place in how care is provided:

- More care—both primary care and related social supports—will be provided in the settings that patients call home, or in their work sites, with an accompanying shift away from delivery of care in physician office and institutional settings. Novel settings in which care may be provided include churches, schools, and grocery stores, and/or by mobile or "pop-up" clinics or kiosks that are linked to hospitals, community health centers, and pharmacies.

- There will be an expansion of novel partnerships to deliver such care, including collaborations among health systems, pharmacies, schools, and community health centers.

- Practitioners will be able to deliver care virtually from anywhere in the world, and to almost anyone in the world with the appropriate internet, cellular, or comparable connection.

- "Uber-like" dispatch systems will enable providers to respond to both urgent and routine care needs; triage patients; send appropriate workers to the home, work site, or other community settings; and assist in coordination of care planning.

- Health care will increasingly be provided in the context of value-based arrangements that link payment to results—either process or outcomes measures, or a combination of both.

- There will be ongoing assessments of work flow in health care settings and in distributed care settings, to ensure that various segments of the health care labor force are allocated appropriately at all times. There will be purposeful and strategic decisions about what jobs and tasks can be handled with technology without compromising quality or patient experience, and related efforts to ensure t will be desirable to have an increasingly nimble pool of workers that responds quickly to changing circumstances.

- New care models will be characterized by widespread task-shifting, in which lower-level workers are educated, trained, and licensed to engage in tasks that were traditionally restricted to higher-level workers, so that humans are not locked into tasks that can be partially, or fully automated. Although it is beyond the scope of this report to describe all new models of care that could be possible in 2025, the Work Force Work Stream selected the following new and evolving models to illustrate how profoundly technology will shape the future health care work force.

The discussion below elaborates on these points, and explicitly discusses the implications for the future health care work force.

- **More care will be provided in the setting that patients call home, or in the work place or other community settings, shifting away from traditional physician office and institutional settings.**

In 2025, the Work Force Work Stream anticipates that the availability of health information and increased access to, and use of, health technology and informatics, will allow patients to receive more high-quality care in non-traditional settings. Under evolving models that focus on delivering care virtually when possible, a wide variety of services and supports could cover most health care episodes that do not require the "laying on of hands" by a clinician. The shift away from providing care exclusively or predominantly in traditional physician office and institutional settings means more care would be provided in apartments, single-family homes, assisted living facilities, and in the homes of adult children with full-time caregiving responsibilities for elderly parents, as well as in schools and work sites.

As technology continues to increase health care workers' access to patients' information in remote locations, as well as a means for real-time, two-way transmission of vital signs and other basic information, patients stand to benefit from more direct connections to the health care system. There will also be new opportunities for health care workers to extend their reach into the community to settings where their patients are most comfortable and likely to benefit from care. For example, Geisinger Health System is already developing a model of "Geisinger at Home," which is built on a Home-Based Medical Care and Community Based Palliative Care program, and which expands Mobile Integrated Health to deliver a spectrum of clinical services at home that help high-cost, complex patients to avoid tertiary settings when possible. The Home-Based Medical Care program uses a care team led by physicians and advanced practitioners that will provide comprehensive and coordinated care to patients with multiple chronic conditions.

Similarly, Mercy Virtual developed an "electronic home kit" to support high-risk Medicare Advantage patients. Patients are taught how to use devices in the kit, and a team of nurses and social workers engages regularly with patients to solve problems, monitor health conditions, and determine when in-person visits are necessary.

In general, then, the implications for the health care work force are these: Health care workers will deliver care in a much wider array of settings using telehealth, mobile, and other technologies, and as a result, they will need to learn how to deliver care in these settings, and how to operate the technologies that are used in these settings. They will also need to be trained in handling the practical challenges they may encounter when delivering care virtually such as poor lighting, or even patients' concerns that care providers will "see" into their homes. For those care providers who visit patients in their homes, logistical issues may arise, such as "walk-up" apartment buildings, or difficulties in parking.

- **There will be expansion of novel partnerships such as collaborations among health systems, payers, employers, pharmacies, school districts, and community health centers, among others.**

As noted in prior chapters of this report, the health care marketplace is changing rapidly, with various new combinations of organizations (among them, CVS and Aetna, and Walmart and Humana, Walgreen's and health systems such as New York Presbyterian) potentially coming together to disrupt and alter current models of health care delivery. There is also considerable untapped capacity in the ability of community-based organizations to partner for improvement of public health on the local level. Under new collaborative arrangements, these organizations are well-suited to "meet people where they are" in the community, and to provide services where they are needed using trusted relationships and local resources.

For example, schools are poised to enhance provision of preventive health care in the pediatric population, pharmacies are positioned to take larger roles in medication management and reduction of medication errors, and community health centers can expand their scope of service provision well beyond periodic health screenings and seasonal vaccination programs. These organizations can work together with local or regional health systems to give communities more options for accessing primary care in non-traditional settings that enjoy a high degree of trust and recognition. Importantly, these novel care settings can be established as permanent venues, or they can be operated as "pop-up" clinics that function on an episodic basis (e.g. in August to provide school physicals) or in response to emergencies such as a natural disaster or disease outbreak.

Through these and other collaborations, diverse segments of the health care work force will forge new working relationships that will ultimately facilitate care provisions and result in better patient outcomes. Under these new partnerships, different types of health care workers will need to develop understanding of their colleagues' roles and contributions to patient health and well-being, and how these colleagues can be engaged to optimize care planning and delivery. In some cases, these new collaborations will involve the need for workers to overcome an historical sense of "competition" with other segments of the health care work force, and to develop respect and appreciation for the contributions of other workers whose roles may have been undervalued in the past.

Health professions schools and other education and training programs, including continuing education, will need to teach their students to work in teams, and to communicate the importance of changes to professional societies and accrediting bodies. Many of these activities are already under way under the auspices of organizations such as the Interprofessional Education Collaborative, which works in collaboration with academic institutions to promote interprofessional education and training, and the Health Professions Accreditors Collaborative, which links organizations that accredit schools of education in medicine, osteopathic medicine, nursing, pharmacy, dentistry, and public health to pursue important developments in interprofessional education.

- **Practitioners will be able to provide care virtually from anywhere in the world.**

The rapid development of health information and technology systems has challenged longstanding notions of what it means for health care providers to be able to access their patients and deliver care, and vice versa. Until recently, a health care provider and a patient needed to be physically together in the same room for a care episode to occur, and such physical visits were typically the only type that could be reimbursed. However, today in many instances, a health care delivery episode consists of a structured exchange of information—physical or virtual—between patients and providers that is supplemented by accessing historical patient information such as blood pressure, weight, or blood glucose measures. With this information, the patient and the provider work together to identify a forward course of action. In the future, patients' health information may increasingly be gathered through such technologies as virtual monitoring and/or digital apps, and patients may also be able to gather additional information via self-administered lab tests.

In 2025, the information that underpins these critical interactions will be able to be obtained by providers from anywhere in the world, as long as a reliable Internet connection is available, and these providers can interact with patients from any location. Patient-provider partnerships will no longer be limited to in-person interactions that must occur in medical office buildings, hospitals, or nursing homes. In many cases, care can be provided virtually anywhere in the world that supports the necessary technology platforms that underpin these important relationships. Clinicians and other providers will be able to support patients in a more flexible manner that is constrained only by their ability to access a computer or other technology, such as a smart phone, that allows them to connect to their patients.

These approaches to care delivery will require providers to become proficient with the technology that enables virtual care provision. They will also need to become proficient with a new set of clinical skills related to the provision of virtual health care, as well as access to, and use of, health informatics to support virtual health care provision. The flexibility associated with virtual health care provision will enable the health care work force to deliver care in ways that are not only more convenient and less expensive for patients and payers, but that also allow providers to be more efficient and effective in reaching larger numbers of patients.

- **"Uber-like" or "Lyft-like" dispatch systems will respond to both urgent and routine care needs, triage patients, and send appropriate workers to the home.**

The rise in popularity of local clinics that provide urgent care and primary care services 24/7 reflects a growing preference on the part of consumers for convenient access to health care services when they are needed, not just during normal business hours. Although these clinics deliver services in brick-and-mortar settings, the recent growth in this type of care delivery parallels growth in consumer preferences for fast-response, custom-tailored services such as those provided by companies like Uber, Amazon, and by many supermarket chains that allow customers to shop online for groceries and have them delivered to the door. Part of the success of these companies and services lies in their ability to respond quickly to their customers' requests, a feature that has become increasingly valued as consumers adopt technology supports to manage basic needs like transportation and shopping.

In 2025, coordinated health care services and supports could be delivered to the home by similar dispatch services. These services could provide both urgent and routine care, and they could leverage information and technology to assess patients' changing needs so that appropriate health care workers and support service providers are sent to the home.

As health care workers begin to deliver care to the home with increasing frequency, they will become linked—ideally in teams—with new entities that will provide triage functions similar to those in traditional hospitals and doctors' offices. These systems will provide an efficient, centralized means for patients to access needed care, and for the health care system to respond to these needs by delivering services to patients, rather than patients delivering themselves to providers. Under this general model, many health care workers will be "dispatched" to community settings in much the same way that emergency workers are dispatched through the 911 system; however, these new delivery systems will include routine primary and preventive care, chronic care management, long-term care supports and services, as well as ancillary services to support nutrition, employment, and other social and economic determinants of health. These types of dispatch systems are going to require many types of health care workers to function in new ways, both in terms of where they deliver care, but also in how the care they provide is administered.

- **New value-based payment arrangements will shift workers from an historical focus on health care "visits," and lead to greater emphasis on how the process of care can achieve favorable health care outcomes.**

Value-based arrangements will give health systems new incentives to partner with others in the community, such as social service agencies, to achieve optimal patient outcomes. Concurrent with these changes, social services and other community-based agencies will contract with health care providers in new community-focused delivery models. Under value-based arrangements, highly integrated care teams comprised of workers from a wide variety of local organizations will work together on behalf of patients and their families to bridge the gap between the health care and social service systems. This new approach to care will be characterized by a greatly diminished focus on individual health care "visits" or "episodes" that address an isolated health problem that is paid for as a distinct unit, and an increase in long-term, multidisciplinary care strategies aimed at treating the "whole person."

These new, value-based arrangements are likely to fundamentally challenge health care workers' historical thinking on what care provision means from a conceptual point of view. The diminished focus on care as an "episode," "visit," or "cost unit" that is provided by a single individual will be accompanied by greater emphasis on long-term processes of care that may involve many types of workers who address a wide variety of inter-related health and social issues, both in the patient's home and in traditional office-based settings. This approach to care will require workers to interact and communicate in new ways with one another, to understand and access data and information in new ways, and to recognize and value the contributions of each member of the team to the overall well-being of the patients for whom they care. Workers will also need to think about receiving payment for their services in ways that depart from historical norms that are based on individual office visits or acute care episodes.

2. New Roles and Expanded Scope of Practice for Existing Health Care Workers

As previously noted in this report, the Work Force Work Stream of the Health Care Without Walls initiative envisions that the evolution of science and technology, coupled with an increasing focus on the social and economic determinants of health, will facilitate profound changes in the roles that are currently played by the existing health care work force. Consider these current trends:

- There is already increased focus on preventive medicine, primary care, and the social determinants of health and the social and economic contexts in which patients live most of their lives. For example, at ProMedica Health System, based in Toledo, Ohio, patients are already screened for basic social determinants needs, such as in housing and transportation, when they enter the system. [130]

- In diseases such as cancer, there is already more focus on precision medicine calibrated to specific genetic characteristics of cancer type. Such advances are generating a groundswell of drug development that will change how many conditions—especially those diseases with a strong genetic component—will be treated in the future. New medications are transforming some cancers that used to require surgical intervention and office-based infusions into conditions that are managed effectively with oral medications that are taken at home.

These trends will only continue, and they will require all elements of the health care work force to evolve and fundamentally alter their care provision strategies in response to changing circumstances. The Work Force Work Stream envisions a future health care system where pharmacists, nurses, and community health workers will assume larger roles as part of diversified health care teams engaging in primary care, chronic disease management, precision medicine, and addressing social and economic determinants of health. Nurses, social workers, pharmacists and pharmacy technicians, home health workers, behavioral health specialists, and other health care workers will function within broadened scopes of practice, and at or near the tops of their licenses.

Care teams will place greater emphasis on efforts to preserve and strengthen psychological and emotional well-being, and to the extent possible, proactively address the social and economic determinants of health. All members of care teams will have distinct roles in optimizing patient access to, and full use of, technology, and these workers will themselves make optimal use of all health information that is available and relevant to care planning.

As a result of all of the changes, there will be an evolution in (1) the tasks in which various segments of the current health care work force will engage in the future; (2) the scope of practice of existing workers and (3) how effort is allocated across categories of workers with respect to job tasks. As noted earlier in this report, as technology performs or streamlines many tasks, there will be a general upward shift in the types of tasks in which health care workers engage. The logical concomitant will be, on the one hand, a move toward working at the top of license, and on the other, increased use of task-shifting. Although physicians will undoubtedly remain at the top of the health care worker hierarchy, their efforts will be concentrated on tasks that can only be completed by them, and even these tasks will be facilitated in new ways by technology. Advance practice nurses, pharmacists, community health workers and possibly other types of health care workers will engage in more clinically-oriented tasks than they do now. These shifts will require many workers to acquire new skills in response to an expanded scope of work, as well as new ways of interacting with physicians or others who will manage the care teams.

Regardless of their backgrounds and training, all clinicians will also need to have a grounding in how to collect, analyze, and apply data and information in a manner that is consistent with their role in patient care. Given the continued digitization of care, clinicians of the future will need a basic understanding of bio-informatics as a core aspect of their digital health skill set. The informatics community has done considerable work in trying to develop core competencies for clinicians of the future,[131] and these types of considerations should be at the forefront of efforts to overhaul health professions' education programs. At the same time, new needs will arise for new types of workers specifically trained in the use and application of data and information (as described further in the next section on new types of workers, below).

Although it is beyond the scope of this report to describe precisely how these technology and other trends will affect the day-to-day roles and scope of practice of all types of health care workers, the remainder of this section describes some of these anticipated changes for several types of health care workers.

Physicians (and in many instances, advanced practice nurses, as discussed further below) will continue evolving toward being lead coordinators of care teams, possibly for panels of patients that are far larger than a typical patient panel today. As part of this continued evolution, primary care physicians will likely interact with a larger variety of health and social service providers than they do today, and these physicians will need to learn and understand the roles and contributions of these workers as part of their leadership and team-building responsibilities. Primary care physicians will also have more e-consults with specialists so that more complex patients will be able to be managed in primary care settings with a corresponding decrease in referrals for specialist visits. Assuming that this trend persists, it may well open up specialists' calendars, thereby reducing wait times for patients seeking care from these providers.

In general, and across medical and surgical practice areas, physicians are likely to engage more in virtual consults, virtual patient visits, and monitoring activities, tasks that will require them to understand these technologies and to work at the top of their specializations. As noted above, for some physicians, care will become even more specialized because of concurrent secular changes in drug development and other factors that are driving the move toward personalized medicine.

For some physicians such as radiologists, much of the workload that is present today may be displaced in the future by technologies like machine-based radiological reading, and these providers will continue to see an increase in the number and amount of services that are provided virtually or through consolidated networks. Radiologists, in particular, offer a useful example of a group of health care workers for which there will likely be dramatic shifts in what tasks will need to be performed, and how these tasks are performed in the future.[132]

As noted in the Technology chapter of this report, the ability to deliver high-resolution digital images over long distances has already resulted in meaningful changes in how radiologists practice. These clinicians no longer need to be onsite where the images are taken, a trend that will likely result in the continuation of current trends, in which images are likely to be recorded in one place and interpreted by radiologists in another.

In addition, as imaging techniques continue to improve, and AI software is developed that can read and interpret films with increased accuracy, it will probably be the case that there will be decreased demand for radiologists to interpret films that software algorithms can identify as having unambiguously negative findings. Instead, these clinicians may concentrate their time on reading films that proven radiology AI software has flagged as being of questionable quality, images that the software suggests may show positive findings, or findings that must be interpreted by a qualified physician for other reasons.

Thus, although the field of radiology is unlikely to disappear, technology will play an increasing role in the process of interpreting radiologic images, thereby shifting the allocation of tasks in which radiologists are likely to engage on a day to day basis. The American College of Radiology—as well as other professional societies, such as pathology, that support health professionals whose roles will be affected by similar changes—will need to think carefully about how to prepare their constituencies for the changes that lie ahead.

Surgeons—particularly surgical specialists—will probably engage in more virtual consults through video-based technologies that are combined with surgical robotics technologies that allow virtual surgeons to work together with local ones who operate on the patient. Surgeons are also likely to work more in tandem with surgical robots, including performing remote surgeries via robots; to train on virtual reality systems; and to train other surgeons in the performance of surgeries virtually.

Advanced practice nurses, including nurse practitioners, certified nurse midwives, certified registered nurse anesthetists, and clinical nurse specialists, will increasingly work at the tops of their licenses and play larger roles on care teams, particularly in provision of primary and preventive care and chronic disease management. These nurses will potentially have more prescribing authority in many states, as well as the ability to work independently without direct physician supervision in hospitals, community-based clinics, and long-term care facilities. They will engage in more telephonic case management as well as high-level care coordination.

Because of the anticipated expansion in their scope of practice, advanced practice nurses will take on numerous new tasks related to basic patient management, a shift that will likely result in delegation of many of their current tasks to medical assistants and similar workers. Like physicians, advance practice nurses will need to become familiar with the technologies and monitoring systems that will be used to provide and track the care they manage, and these professionals will need to develop more supervisory and management skills than they currently use in routine practice.

Registered nurses will also assume larger roles in care delivery, especially in primary care. Although they will continue to have a different scope of practice than advanced practice nurses, registered nurses will nonetheless play a much larger role in new primary care delivery models, such as patient-centered medical homes.

Pharmacists will play larger roles in multidisciplinary care teams, particularly for the care of complex patients requiring polypharmacy to manage multiple chronic health conditions. It is also likely that pharmacists may receive prescribing authority in some states, some circumstances, and for some conditions (e.g. uncomplicated urinary tract or ear infections), especially in settings where a brick-and-mortar pharmacy contains a clinic that is staffed by a nurse with prescribing authority.

Pharmacists are also likely to expand their presence as members of care teams in terms of medication management efforts, and by acting in consulting and supportive capacities to various members of the care team. Others are likely to focus on enhanced management for patients with five or more medications because these patients are most prone to medication errors and challenges with adherence. Many of these efforts will also take place virtually. For example, SinfoníaRx, a company established in 2006 at the University of Arizona College of Pharmacy, provides customizable medication therapy management services remotely to patients—typically in their own homes—through relationships with health plans, pharmacy benefit managers, community pharmacies, colleges of pharmacy, and clinical practices. There is little reason why such remotely-provided medication management therapy services should not become standard for chronically ill patients in the future.

Pharmacists are also likely to expand their role as educators and "coaches" for patients. For example, some pharmacists are also becoming Certified Diabetes

Educators, an example of a "stackable credential" that can be added to other qualifications over time as a professional moves along a career pathway.

In the future, such changes may be propelled forward further by an increase in moves to make certain medications—such as statins—available on an over-the-counter basis, or by the availability of "behind-the-counter" medications—commonly used, non-narcotic drugs that are currently only available by prescription, but that may be available in the future through structured consultations between a patient and pharmacist. If such changes in the pharmaceuticals marketplace do take place, pharmacists are likely to be in greater need than ever for one-on-one consultations, either physical or virtual.

In areas with relatively scant access to good primary care, community pharmacists in particular could be well positioned to play expanded roles along these lines. A large recent survey showed that a community pharmacy model that incorporated an integrated health electronic record system, a comprehensive level of point-of-care diagnostic testing, and some physical examination procedures would be attractive to patients, payers, and community pharmacists alike.[133] New care models that linked family practice physicians with community pharmacists, and that marshalled pharmacists' skills to provide preventive care, teach patients self-management techniques, and collaboration with physicians and other clinicians on chronic disease management, could be particularly important additions to the health care landscape in rural and other underserved areas.

Social workers currently have established roles in hospitals and other settings, but these roles also are likely to expand in the future. Advances in technology will have a particular impact on hospital-based social workers because of their central role in discharge planning. A key feature of the new models of care that were described earlier in this report is enhanced coordination among community-based resources and supports, and increased use of social, behavioral, and health-related data in team-based care planning. At the point of hospital discharge, social workers will not only continue to facilitate patient access to community-based resources, they will also be instrumental in setting the stage for these patients to optimize technology supports in the recovery process. As "Hospital at Home" programs expand, social workers are also likely to play important roles in coordinating and ensuring the availability of the various social supports that patients need.

Community health workers are likely to join physicians, nurses, pharmacists, and social workers in playing critical roles in care teams. In their expanded roles, these workers will formalize linkages with community-based social support services to bridge the longstanding gap between the clinical and social/economic aspects of health. (See the box on the Ohio State University College of Nursing's programs on p. 209, for an example of how such workers are being trained to combat problems such as infant mortality.)

As the ambiguity around their education, training, certification, and licensure is sorted out, community health workers will engage routinely with patients, their families, and a wide variety of home-based technologies to ensure that the needs of the "whole patient" are recognized and addressed. These workers will be on the front line of service coordination and provision, with an expanded skill set that includes training patients on technology use, patient education, ensuring social connectedness, and identification of new or shifting risk factor profiles. These tasks will require proficiency with data entry and management tasks, as well as ongoing responsibilities focused on assessment of evolving patient and family needs. (Further discussion about training and certification of community health workers is below.)

The home health, home care, and so-called "direct care" work force consists of a broad array of workers who provide health care services or various types of supportive care in the home. This segment of the health care work force includes licensed workers who deliver clinically-oriented services such as medication management and physical therapy, as well as unlicensed workers who help with such non-medical tasks related to the "activities of daily living," such as feeding, dressing, and toileting, as well as with the "instrumental activities of daily living," such as shopping for groceries, which allow people to live independently in their communities.

As the U.S. population continues to age and become more disabled, it is anticipated that the demand for these workers will increase significantly. Technologies, such as robots, may be able to supplant some tasks, and even facilitate maintenance of independence in the community by disabled individuals for longer periods of time than was possible in the past. It is also possible that the broad group of home health care and direct care workers will be employed by health systems, and hybrid medical and social systems such as the Programs of All-Inclusive Care for the Elderly (PACE), as new care coordination strategies continue to develop. Given the widely divergent levels of education and training that direct care workers currently receive, there will clearly be a need to raise these levels to equip such workers for the greater responsibilities they will have and the increased demands that will be made on them—particularly as they are called upon to interact more with technologies.

3. **Task shifting among current types of health care workers**

The Work Force Work Stream emphasized the importance of distinguishing between changes that may occur in the numbers and distribution of different categories of health care jobs, and changes that may occur in specific tasks that various categories of health care workers routinely perform. This section examines how the specific tasks in which health care workers engage may change in response to evolving technology and other factors.

The Work Force Work Stream agreed that there will a growing trend to move selected tasks down the health care job ladder. That is, workers in lower-level jobs will increasingly take on certain tasks that were once done only by higher-level workers. As noted above, this concept, often called "task-shifting," has been described by the World Health Organization (WHO) as, "...a process of delegation whereby tasks are moved, where appropriate, to less specialized health workers." In some developing countries, the training of lower-level workers to deliver more complex and demanding aspects of care arose in large part from the limited supply of physicians and higher-level health care workers, and the need to respond to local circumstances, such as the HIV epidemic.

The WHO has summarized the advantages of task shifting: "By reorganizing the workforce in this way, task shifting presents a viable solution for improving health care coverage by making more efficient use of the human resources already available and by quickly increasing capacity while training and retention programmes [sic] are expanded."[134] However, for task-shifting to be safe, efficient, effective, and sustainable, the WHO notes that critical system-level requirements must be in place. These include an enabling regulatory framework, quality assurance, appropriate supervision, and standardized training, among other elements.[135]

Although the Work Force Work Stream recognizes the fundamental differences between the health care landscape in the U.S. and that in developing countries, it also pointed out a number of similarities that are driving task-shifting in the U.S. Two examples are the need to respond to the maldistribution of health care workers in rural areas, and the need to better position the health care workforce to respond to "local circumstances," such as the aging of the American population. It is well-documented that the supply of primary care physicians rises with the likelihood that a physician's office location is in an urban setting. In rural areas, there are 39.8 primary care physicians per 100,000 population, a figure that rises to 53.3 per 100,000 in urban areas.[136] Rather than train more physicians and persuade them to settle in rural areas, it may be more effective to greatly enhance existing efforts to promote primary care delivery in these areas by advanced practice nurses, registered nurses, and physician assistants, as appropriate.

Although these professionals have worked side-by-side with supervising physicians in ambulatory care settings for years—and in some areas these professionals are already established primary care providers—additional efforts aimed at task-shifting would involve a movement for these professionals to assume increased responsibility for managing more patients, or more complex patients over the long term, perhaps with supervision from offsite primary care physicians as needed. In this example, the scaffolding for task-shifting is already in place, but it could be greatly expanded in the future. This could occur in a targeted effort to enhance primary care delivery in rural and other underserved areas, but it could also involve a far-reaching effort to shift routine primary care provision from physicians to nurses or physician assistants across the board.

A second example of how task-shifting could benefit the U.S. health care system is that it could help prepare the country to meet the current and future needs of an aging society. The scaffolding for task-shifting in this setting is less well-developed than it is in rural primary care delivery. The national shortage of geriatricians comes at a time when these specialists are most needed to handle the complex medical profiles of increasing numbers of older adults.[137] Virtual care modalities such as telehealth could in effect leverage the skills and knowledge of the comparatively small number of geriatricians, while less highly trained workers took on other aspects of care delivery to geriatric patients.

In addition to the shortage of geriatric physician-specialists, there is also a shortage of professionals who are licensed to provide routine medical support in the home, such as medication dispensing, checking vital signs, and interacting with the patient's primary care provider. Currently, home health nurses often provide these services. In geriatric care, task-shifting could involve training these home health nurses to assume a greater role for overall care management, as well as training home health aides to take on tasks such as medication management and collection and documentation of vital signs—tasks typically reserved for home health nurses. These and other task shifts could be facilitated by technologies such as virtual connections to supervisors and readily available electronic health records at the point of service. In this way, task-shifting could not only help fill key gaps in the health care work force, it could also provide lower- to mid-level workers with more responsibility, enhanced skills, and potentially greater job satisfaction.

Although there are many other examples of how and where task-shifting could occur in the U.S. health care system, it is beyond the scope of this report to describe them all. However, the Work Force Work Stream emphasized that continued technological innovation, combined with changing demographics, evolving patient preferences, and ongoing cost pressures, will likely continue to drive task-shifting in the future. If task shifting is to be encouraged, health systems and others will also need to examine pay and benefits structures, and potentially "sharing the wealth:" shifting more pay and benefits to workers who have historically been less well paid, as they take on tasks once performed by higher-paid workers.

4. **New Types of Health Care Workers**

As noted, the Work Force Work Stream envisions that ongoing advances in health and information technology, combined with new ways of providing care, will result in the need for new types of health care workers. Many of these workers either do not exist in our current system, or components of the work they would perform may be reflected in existing job titles, and may need to be consolidated and formalized under new job titles and functions that reflect the health care landscape of the future. In some organizations, the "new jobs" that are described in this section may not be new at all; the tasks described as needing to be performed by workers may already be performed currently, but under differently configured positions than those described below.

Whatever the case, to fully employ technology and health informatics, a targeted effort is needed to define the new health care jobs and tasks that will be needed in the future. New models of care, continued innovations in health technology and informatics, and a shift toward provision of care in homes and in the community, will all drive the need to formally develop, educate, and train new types of health care workers. Participants expressed the belief that many of these new positions and types of workers may either augment, or may supplant, existing types of workers, and echoed concerns that if they merely augmented the health care work force, they may contribute to health care's productivity problems and cost disease. The work stream emphasized that it would be important for new payment models to create maximum incentives to employ these new types of workers efficiently, perhaps through capitation or more global payment models.

Regardless, the Work Force Work Stream concurred that there will be a need for health care workers to fill roles that either do not exist today, or a need to fill existing roles that must be re-imagined to such a large extent that they essentially become new jobs. These new workers will need to be integrated into a fast-paced, ongoing process that also involves profound changes in the existing health care work force as well as continued advances in technology. These new workers will likely become identified with new or existing professional associations, and in turn, these organizations will play important roles in providing education, training, and certification and licensure to these new workers.

There are obvious challenges associated with exploring specific features of new types of health care workers that do not currently exist in the formal sense. Despite these challenges, the Work Force Work Stream identified several new job types that will become critical under a re-imagined health care system. It is important to emphasize that these *new jobs* are distinct from the *new tasks* for which existing health care workers may become responsible in the future, as discussed in the previous section. This section, by contrast, defines some of the new types of health care workers that will be needed to meet the Health Care Without Walls vision for 2025; provides examples of tasks for which these workers will be responsible; and describes how they will interact with other workers as well as various types of health and information technology.

Some of the new types of workers, and their responsibilities, that the work stream foresaw include the following:

Medical "Virtualist"

As noted in a recent report[138] in the *Journal of the American Medical Association*, there has been marked growth in non-procedural health care that is being provided virtually through telemedicine technologies. This growth has been driven by changing consumer preferences, the availability of new technology platforms, and new businesses that support these services. Virtual care is being provided in parallel with increased use of health technologies such as home blood pressure and glucose monitoring equipment, as well as increased use of home-based sensors that can monitor gait, balance, sleep, and other factors that provide important insight into health and well-being.

The many sources of health information are driving the need to develop physician competencies to access, manage, and act on this wealth of information. As noted in the *JAMA* report, "The coordination of virtual care with home visits, virtual monitoring, and simultaneous family engagement is changing the perception and reality of virtual health care." In response to this changing reality, the authors of the JAMA report argue, medical virtualists will be needed.

As described in the *JAMA* report, these professionals will spend most, or all, of their time providing virtual patient care, including providing leadership to, and coordinating, multidisciplinary teams that offer both in-office and virtual care. Because such physicians will spend the majority or all of their time caring for patients using a virtual medium, they will require a "set of core competencies to be further developed over time."[139]

However, it remains to be seen whether such a position will indeed evolve, or whether virtual care will simply become a routine care modality that all physicians and clinicians will routinely engage in, with competency-based training and education eventually integrated into all curriculums. At Kaiser Permanente, for example, physicians engage in both virtual and physical visits, and many physicians believe they benefit from seeing patients in both types of settings. It may simply be that, regardless of how much of their time is spent in virtual care provision, physicians along with other types of clinicians will need to be trained, and demonstrate competency in, conducting virtual medical visits and delivering care using telemedicine and other virtual technologies. They will also need to demonstrate competencies in management and acting on patient health data obtained from diverse sources (e.g. virtual monitoring devices, electronic medical records, pharmacy records), and in using this information to coordinate the delivery of services by the care teams they supervise.

Chief Information/Technology Officer, Health System Level

Although it is likely that the amount and complexity of health- and health-care related data that will be collected in the future will continue to increase, it is not likely that any individual clinician will have the time, inclination, or ability, to access, manage, or synthesize this enormous volume of data, let alone to understand and apply these data for informed health care decision-making. The existing core of individuals within health systems who today are known as chief information or chief clinical officers will have new responsibilities in the realm of collecting, synthesizing and analyzing these data, and putting actionable information in front of clinicians and care teams.

These individuals are likely to oversee entire departments composed of, for example, other health information and technology systems specialists and managers, who would be responsible for the design, maintenance, and ongoing upgrading of system-level technologies that support the new care delivery systems described earlier in this report. These workers will be responsible for ensuring that patient information from diverse sources is integrated and accessible by all members of the care team. Examples of systems that are moving in this direction are Kaiser Permanente; the Mayo Clinic; and the Geisinger health system, among others.

Health Information and Technology System Specialist

In addition to the position of chief technology/information officer within health systems, there will be increasing needs for other individuals who work at high levels within these systems and take various responsibilities for the design, maintenance, and ongoing upgrading of system-level technologies that support the new care delivery systems that will be developed in the future.

Health Information and Technology Technician

In the near future, the health care landscape will be characterized by increased delivery of services and supports to the home and other community settings, routine interactions between patients and providers using online platforms, and increased use of passive, home-based sensors, Wi-Fi-enabled active monitoring devices, and other health technologies. In this new landscape, patients will need technologies deployed in their homes, work sites, and other distributed settings. They will also need the support to set up the technology, learn to use it, troubleshoot when problems arise, and modify the functionality in response to changing circumstances.

It is therefore likely that individuals will need to be employed by health systems and provider organizations, or potentially by a health plan, to be deployed to homes or other community settings to assist patients and families with these concerns. These technicians could engage in tasks such as ensuring that patients have adequate internet access to support the functionality of their medical devices; teaching patients, as well as formal and informal caregivers, how to operate their devices; and also educating patients in their caregivers on how to access their online information and communicate with the provider team using online portals. These new workers would also be available by phone to field troubleshooting calls, and they could be re-deployed to patient homes to adjust equipment, change settings, or to remove equipment when a patient's condition no longer required use of a specific device.

Health and Wellness Liaison

In 2025, a health and wellness liaison could be responsible for helping patients and families optimize their access to, and use of, services and supports not only for health, but if needed, also for housing, food, and employment. This role could be that of a technology-enabled, clinically-focused extension of a traditional case manager. In many cases, health and wellness liaisons would work as part of a multidisciplinary care team that could be managed largely or entirely by a medical virtualist.

These individuals would be tech-savvy, have access to patient information, and they would be familiar with local resources, including supports and services that are outside traditional medical care, such as food and transportation. The health and wellness liaison would work closely with community health workers to help connect families with needed services, and they would also report back to the care team with information about social and environmental factors that may influence patients' health, and what steps are being taken to address these health determinants.

Robots and Robotic Technologies

The Work Force Work Stream emphasized the enduring importance of human interactions in the provision of health care, but it also acknowledged that robots and robotic technologies are currently being used to perform various tasks in some care settings. There is little doubt that the breadth of the tasks that robots perform will only increase in the future. It is for this reason that robots are examined as a new type of worker in this report.

Robots are currently used in some larger hospitals for tasks such as stocking medications, delivering goods, and packing sterile supplies. As the cost of robotic technologies decreases, more hospitals will be able to afford these in-house labor supports. In addition, the number of tasks that robots can effectively complete will increase in the future to include more automated packing functions, more applications for use in surgical procedures, greeting and lifting patients, and for virtual monitoring in the ICU and other high-risk inpatient settings.[140,141]

Aside from having robots perform these more readily automated tasks, there is growing evidence that patients around the world are willing to receive certain types of health care from robots, including those equipped with augmented intelligence capabilities, if that care is associated with better access, fast and accurate diagnosis, and if it does not completely replace human interaction.[142] It is therefore likely that robots or robotic technologies will be increasingly utilized for certain applications linked to diagnosis and care.

Some interactive robotic technologies are designed to alleviate loneliness through social interaction with patients, either when accessed virtually, or when deployed in the home. Other companion robots provide mobility assistance in the home and analyze the home environment, so they can effectively monitor the individuals who live there. As America's population continues to age, it is likely that robots or robotic technologies will also be used to provide social support and interaction for older, isolated adults.

5. **Potential job displacement and re-allocation of effort**

As noted throughout this report, advances in technology, changes in scope of practice, and expanded application of AI into the health care sector will undoubtedly result in reduced work force needs in some fields or occupations, and increased demand in others. Although it is certain that these changes will occur—they are already happening—there is considerable uncertainty about the extent of these changes, which professions will be affected, to what degree, and in which direction.

Some of the uncertainty in anticipating the extent of re-allocation of various segments of the health care work force stems from the rapid pace of technological change, the ongoing evolution of new models of care, and potentially influential changes in how health care is financed. Despite these uncertainties, the Work Force Work Stream agreed that it was important to offer a framework for thinking about how technology and information/informatics will play into anticipated changes for various health care providers, and to provide some perspective on this complex issue.

Concerns about the role of technology in driving reductions in demand for health care workers—especially the potential for reduced demand for physicians—are often raised in relation to the rise of AI, and what role these and other technologies will play in the future of health care delivery. Above, this report cited radiology as an example of how AI is already changing demand for radiology services, and it provides a model for how AI may impact other clinical disciplines that rely heavily on objective data for clinical decision-making. In the radiology example, AI technologies are likely to play an increasing role in providing preliminary interpretation of routine radiographic images, with radiologists potentially focused on interpretation of clinically challenging or ambiguous images and low-quality images, or on new tasks such as providing quality control and clinical oversight for radiology software development and maintenance, including any updates that may be needed in response to new knowledge in the field.

The growing use of telestroke and telepsychiatry services in emergency departments offer additional examples of how technology may impact the demand and allocation of physician labor in the future. Stroke patients often present in emergency departments where immediate assessment is critical for patient outcomes.

Yet rapid access to neurologists with expertise in stroke management can be challenging, especially in rural areas and low-volume hospitals. Emergency departments also have millions of mental health and substance abuse visits each year, yet it often takes many hours to access a psychiatrist to evaluate patients with critical needs.

These delays often have an unfavorable impact on the patient, and they are also costly to the hospital. Although *locum tenens,* or temporary coverage by replacement providers, may offer one solution to some of these challenges, this choice may be less cost-effective for hospitals if they can access qualified neurologists, psychiatrists and other specialists through contractual arrangements with telehealth providers that connect them with the physicians they need with little or no delay. In fact, in 2018, Geisinger Health System in central Pennsylvania is recruiting urologists in metropolitan areas who can assist in providing telehealth visits to Geisinger patients. In a similar care delivery model, one or a few virtual specialists can support the needs of many hospital emergency departments or primary care physicians, thereby reducing, but not eliminating the need to have specialists physically present in these settings.

Physicians are unlikely to be the only health professionals who will experience changes in the demand for labor, or for whom tasks evolve in response to changing circumstances. There are likely to be corresponding changes for advance practice nurses, pharmacists, home health aides, and community health workers. Increasing use of virtual care may allow the health care system a new form of flexibility in utilizing its labor resources.

An analogy could be drawn to the supply of, and demand for, electricity, and how it is managed by adjustments in the electrical grid. Electric power can be re-allocated across this system in response to changing demand. Similarly, when more care is provided virtually, this labor supply could be routed across the country to areas of greatest demand—for example, from cities to rural areas, or even from one part of the country to another to take time differences into account. Under such an arrangement, West Coast providers working their normal business hours could be martialed to serve after-hours consumer needs on the East Coast. In effect, technology could enable health care work force reallocation to facilitate access to care when and where it is needed, thereby optimizing workforce utility and efficiency.

Overall, the Work Force Work Stream agreed that technology will drive marked changes in the demand for various job categories, with a reduction or re-allocation for some types of jobs, and corresponding increases for others as they assume new tasks linked to increased scope of practice, coupled with adoption of new technologies. However, the group emphasized that details concerning how this would play out for specific segments of the health care labor market remain unclear.

6. Evolving Employer-Employee Relationships

In addition to reallocation of labor, task-shifting, and increased flexibility in using the labor supply, the very nature of how health care workers are "attached" to their employers is evolving. Historically, health care workers had a single employer, and this attachment was linked to job-related elements as varied as promotions, vacation accrual, retirement benefits, and weekly scheduling. Because many workers no longer need to be closely connected to a physical location, the traditional link between job and "work place" has begun to erode.

In addition, according to large health systems such as Geisinger, increasing numbers of health care workers are responding to the growing popularity of the "gig economy" by seeking multiple part-time or contractual arrangements instead of a traditional, full-time job. By their nature, telehealth companies, health systems, and providers of other types of virtual health care are not constrained by a specific building or buildings or a 40-hour work week; clinicians who deliver care in these settings can theoretically work for as many delivery organizations as their schedules can handle. These ways of working may introduce new worker-employer relationships into health care, and raise basic questions concerning who the employer is, and who if anyone is responsible for employee benefits. Other, more subtle questions such as those relating to organizational commitment and loyalty on the part of the future health care workforce have also been raised.

As health care provider systems, professional societies, and other organizations begin to grapple with these changes, it will be important for them and their constituencies to be proactive about understanding how jobs and tasks will change, and positioning workers to be nimble and responsive to these changes. This includes ensuring that the existing health care work force has access to necessary re-training, that degree programs and curricula meet the needs of future students, and that continuing education, licensure and certification closely reflect the skills that are needed in response to changes in tasks and job responsibilities. The Work Force Work Stream agreed that health care stakeholders who are responsible for education and training will need to remain especially adaptable to changing circumstances to ensure that their constituencies acquire and maintain the skills that are needed in this rapidly-changing landscape.

7. Updated Education and Training

In light of the other elements of the multi-part framework—new care models, new roles and expanded scope of practice for existing types of health care workers, the opportunities for task shifting, the development of new types of health care workers, and the likelihood of job displacement—the Work Force Work Stream envisioned that bold changes will be needed in the final element of the framework: health care education and training.

There was agreement that the current work force contains a talented pool of workers with tremendous potential to meet the needs of the technology-enabled, distributed health care system envisioned for 2025. However, the Work Force Work Stream also expressed the conviction that, at the current time, these workers do not have the training and skills that will be needed to optimize technology offerings in 2025, nor do they have the team-based skills that will be required to deliver the coordinated, multidisciplinary care that is envisioned in the future. In addition, the group pointed out that trends that are driving the development of a more distributed health care system will result in the shuffling and re-allocation of existing roles, with some types of existing workers being in higher demand, while the need for other types of workers will diminish. This shuffling of roles will require existing workers to obtain new skills that reflect the demands of their new roles.

Finally, as discussed above, new types of workers will emerge in the future health care landscape. These workers must have clearly-defined roles and responsibilities that are driven by skills-based competencies. In turn, these skills and competencies need to be obtained in new education and training programs.

As a result, the work stream anticipated that (1) new skills will be needed among existing health care workers; (2) existing degree programs will need to be overhauled to reflect advances in technology and changes in how care is delivered, and (3) new certification, degree, and continuing education and training programs will be needed for the new types of workers that will be needed in the future. Recognizing these imperatives will allow community colleges, institutions of higher learning, professional societies, and accrediting bodies to plan high-quality education and training programs for these new health workers, to attract students to new programs, and to strategically deploy graduates into the future health care labor market.

In general, the work stream further grouped the changes needed into the categories listed below:

- Institutions and organizations will need to overhaul existing degree programs to reflect advances in technology and new models of care. Here again, the OSU College of Nursing is an example of an institution that has added telehealth education to its curriculum for both graduate and undergraduate degrees (see box, below).

- Institutions and organizations will need to provide opportunities for faculty development in technology use and instruction within teaching institutions.

- Institutions and organizations will need to increase integration of technology and informatics into curricula, and improve how technology is taught, with a focus on setting targets for the development of skills and competencies.

- Institutions and organizations will need to increase emphasis on teaching team-based care, and in particular, in virtual contexts.
- Institutions and organizations will need to create new certification and degree programs for new types of health care workers.

- Institutions and organizations will need to formalize titles, roles, and tasks of new jobs, but also think carefully about how tasks and jobs may evolve over time and how to maximize opportunities for a flexible and adaptive work force.

- Institutions and organizations will need to integrate efforts among professional societies, institutions of higher education, community colleges, and online education platforms to develop and deploy curricula to educate and train these new types of workers.

- Institutions and organizations will need to provide practical opportunities for existing workers to become more skilled in the use and application of health information and technology.

- Institutions and organizations will need to devise new continuing education programs, or revise existing ones, to place greater emphasis on technology-enabled and team-based care. The Ohio State University College of Nursing, for example, is creating online, self-paced continuing education materials for a variety of health care providers, including nurse practitioners, registered nurses, and physician assistants.

The Work Force Work Stream also identified several overarching strategies that will help meet the emerging education and training needs of the future health care work force. These include the following:

- Attempts should be made to define new competencies that some or all types of health care workers should have in the future to deliver more virtual care. These should include defining and normalizing new, technology-enriched competencies such as data collection, analysis, synthesis, and application, for each category of health professional, and matching those competencies with skills-based training.

- Attempts should be made to define new categories of workers who will be needed, or to define how existing categories of workers should evolve to meet a changing health care environment.

- New collaborations should be undertaken between degree-granting institutions and academic and professional societies that focus on building technology- and informatics-focused competencies.

- Non-profit organizations and local social service providers should be incorporated into professional education and training.

- The availability of, and access to online education, continuing education, and certification, should increase.

The balance of this section describes key concepts related to health care workers' education and training that will be needed to meet the 2025 vision of a more distributed and technology-enabled health care environment. Specific recommendations concerning how to make these education- and training-related concepts into reality can be found at the end of this report.

Build new skills among existing workers

The Work Force Work Stream emphasized that strategies to define new skills and competencies, and develop them among health care professionals currently in practice, are distinct from the ones that are needed for current and future health care professions students in degree programs. They are also different from those that are needed for new degree and certification programs that will be developed in the future.

Existing health care workers are accustomed to their current workflows, and they may therefore be less inclined to easily adopt new technologies or decision-support strategies. These workers may have also received their initial education and training at a time before the Internet and mobile technologies were available or widely used. Compared to younger workers for whom social norms and facility with technology have been defined during the Internet Age, mid-career and senior-level health professionals may have different sensibilities and comfort levels concerning the importance of face-to-face contact in care provision, working with hardware, software and electronic data, the appropriateness of relying on artificial intelligence and other technological innovations, and whether technology adoption will threaten their jobs or patient-provider relationships.

In addition to these overarching considerations, there are sector-specific issues to consider when contemplating how to build the necessary skills and competencies that will allow current workers to optimize technology in their jobs. For example, practicing physicians will need training in collection, management, and synthesis of electronic data, and how this information can be used to inform better decision-making in the context of team-based care. Even if they eventually work in health systems in which others carry out many of these responsibilities, physicians will need to understand in principle how data collected from many sources will ultimately inform their medical practice.

At the other extreme, home health aides, certified nursing assistants, and similar workers may need re-training in a smaller number of information- and technology-related tasks, but this training would undoubtedly need to include incorporating into their practice data that is compiled from different sources and put to use in diverse care settings. These workers would also need to learn how to engage in tasks such as virtually implementing real-time care planning instructions from a physician or nurse team leader, and how to interact in new ways with other members of the care team.

Although the new skills that will be needed by various sectors of the existing health care work force will differ significantly across sector, they will all have a strong focus on skills-based competencies. Examples of the practical skills that existing health care workers will need to master include the following:

- Learning the practical value of team-based care and applying it in routine practice.

- Developing a working knowledge of health information and technology and how these assets are used in daily decision-making and care delivery.

- Overcoming the practical challenges associated with delivering care outside of traditional brick-and-mortar settings.

- Learning to forge new relationships with non-traditional partners such as schools, senior housing providers, and social service agencies.

- Developing data management and analytic skills that are consistent with job roles so that each type of health care worker can optimize its contribution to patient care.

Although a description of all strategies that could be used to develop new skills among existing workers is beyond the scope of this report, the Work Force Work Stream offers some examples of re-training and skills updating approaches that could be implemented in the future. In many cases, these examples could be re-tooled for use in re-training multiple health worker categories, as follows:

- Collaborate with accreditation bodies and professional societies to embed informatics training into conferences and continuing education.

- Develop new opportunities for continuing education in team-based care.

- Maximize technology and data in the practice environment among clinical faculty who are actively treating patients and teaching students.

- Conduct a comprehensive overhaul of certification and licensure requirements to reflect new competencies in health technology and information that will be taught across the health professions. Examples could include training existing home health aides on motivational interviewing, how to recognize risk factors, and how to teach patients how to use home-based technologies; and training physicians on how to conduct virtual health care visits, how to lead team-based care, and how community resources can be leveraged to enhance care planning.

- Emphasize the creation of, and accumulation by members of the health care work force, of "stackable" credentials in virtual care delivery: i.e., certificates that can be obtained for training to be added on top of an existing degree, or the reverse—courses and skills added to an already-obtained certificate in order to earn a degree. For example, a certificate in virtual care delivery could be added to an advanced practice nursing degree, or a pathway to a master's in health informatics could be created for people who have already obtained a training certificate.

Update existing degree programs to reflect advances in technology and new models of care

Unlike existing health care workers who may have completed their education, the next generation of health professionals should be able to rely on their education and training to provide them with the skills needed to meet the 2025 health care vision. However, the Work Force Work Stream noted that for the most part, the curricula of existing degree programs are not yet adequate to the task. Although some degree programs may offer exposure to team-based care and how health and information technologies are used in daily care delivery, in virtually all cases, these curricular elements are not required for institutional accreditation.

In response to these degree programs' shortcomings in the realms of technology and informatics, the Work Force Work Stream recommended specific steps, as follows:

- Decreasing the gap between competencies that are required for degree programs and skills that are required for real-world care delivery in more virtual settings.

- Developing core competencies in technology and informatics that are appropriate for each type of health professional.

- Promoting understanding of the need to include technology and informatics in curricula and providing opportunities for faculty to develop competencies in teaching in these areas.

- Identifying and promoting thought leaders in different health professions who can act as "curriculum development champions" and communicate the rationale and vision for curricular changes.

- Working with professional societies and accrediting bodies to develop standard curricular elements or modules that can be easily integrated into existing degree and certification programs.

- Increasing the integration of technology into curricula, such as teaching medical students how to conduct a virtual health care visit, and teaching home health aides how to access electronic health records and update information.

- Developing a skills-based approach to technology training that is tailored to the new roles that of each type of health professional will play in the future health care landscape.

- Increasing emphasis on inter-professional education that teaches team-based care, including how it can be delivered in the home and other community settings, and updating curricula to emphasize common core elements.

- Developing curricula, and teaching about how community-based resources such as pharmacies, as well as social services and supports should be considered and integrated into holistic care planning and delivery.

- Defining common curricula and core competencies for high-demand roles such as community health workers and home health aides. Formalizing online and hybrid education programs (some virtual and some classroom or site-based training) for high-demand roles, and enhancing access to these educational offerings through open online courses and community colleges.

Create new certification and degree programs for new types of health care workers

As noted above, new types of health professionals will need to be formally recognized and trained to meet the evolving needs of America's changing health care landscape. The fast pace of technology innovation, coupled with the continued evolution of new models of care creates practical challenges for identifying the types of new workers that are needed, and how they should be educated and trained. With these uncertainties in mind, the Work Force Work Stream identified several types of new workers that it believes will be in high demand in the future. Although it is not possible to lay out a comprehensive strategy describing how each of the new types of workers should be developed in the future, the *JAMA* report[138] on medical virtualists, referenced above, provides a framework for thinking about how to approach this important process.

The *JAMA* report envisioned that medical virtualists will be physicians who are specially trained, and who provide most, or nearly all care through virtual platforms. These physicians could also serve as leads for multidisciplinary teams that provide care through a combination of virtual and traditional, in-person or office-based care episodes. The report offered a framework for training and certification of these professionals:

"Medical virtualists will need specific core competencies and curricula that are beginning to develop at some institutions. In addition to the medical training for a specific discipline, the curriculum for certification should include knowledge of legal and clinical limitations of virtual care, competencies in virtual examination using the patient or families, "virtual visit presence training," inclusion of on-site clinical measurements, as well as continuing education. It will be necessary for early adopters, thought leaders, medical specialty societies, and medical trade associations to work with the certifying organizations to formalize curriculum, training, and certification for medical virtualists. If advances in technology continue and if rigorous evidence demonstrates that this technology improves care and outcomes and reduces cost, medical virtualists could be involved in a substantial proportion of health care delivery for the next generation."[138]

As noted above, there is disagreement over whether a specific new class of "virtualists" will emerge, or whether all physicians and other clinicians, including advanced practice nurses and doctors of pharmacy, will alternate between physical and virtual encounters and must thus be trained in both. There also could be reasonable debate over whether, if there are virtualists, that they should be physicians only, or whether the skills of virtualists will need to exist broadly across multiple types of providers.

A related issue is how some roles in a re-imagined and reconfigured health care environment will need to evolve and be integrated into the new landscape. For example, community health workers currently play a vital role in connecting patients with health care and social services in their communities, and frequently work on teams in various health care settings as well. In these contexts, the use of community health workers can yield improved outcomes.[143] However, these workers are not fully recognized and embedded in health care, in part because the system has been slow to recognize the importance of addressing the social determinants of health, or the community contexts in which patients live most of their lives.

For this portion of the work force to become widely accepted members of the current and future health care team, it will be necessary to build on the existing evidence base, and gain broader recognition, of community health workers' abilities to positively affect patients' outcomes.[144] It will also be necessary to spread knowledge about the ways that community health workers have been integrated successfully into a variety of health care settings. In recent years, important efforts to train and educate community health workers have been developed at such institutions as the University of Pennsylvania and the Ohio State University College of Nursing. In the case of the Ohio State program, a critical goal is to produce more such workers to help address a high regional infant mortality rate and major disparities in care outcomes for African-Americans.

It may also be necessary to require more consistency around the definition of what constitutes a community health worker. The role of community health workers, typically as unlicensed care providers, is not fully characterized, and varies greatly based on the setting in which they work. There is an ongoing debate in many quarters about whether community health workers should be credentialed and licensed, as with other health professionals, or whether such measures would fundamentally change the nature of an occupation with its roots as peer promotores/promotoras—promoters of health—especially in Latino communities. As a result, only a few states, such as Minnesota, currently have credentialing programs and requirements for these workers. Many employers of community health workers provide direct training for them on the job, but there is no broadly accepted or recognized education and training curriculum for them.

In addition to educating licensed care professionals on community health workers' roles and impact, community health workers will undoubtedly need training to help them practice at the top of their capacity. They will also need training to employ new technology tools. Currently, there is a movement under way to create a national organization for community health workers to promote greater understanding of their unique roles through a uniform set of skills and competencies.[145] With increasingly high demand for community health worker services, such an organization could provide a foundational element for this profession to be formally recognized and integrated as a critical role in the future health care work force.

> **HEALTH CARE WITHOUT WALLS AT OHIO STATE**
>
> The Ohio State University College of Nursing, based in the state capital Columbus and with regional campuses throughout Ohio, has fully embraced the notion that the "Health Care

Without Walls" movement will reshape both health care delivery and education for health care professionals. "We want to be the world's leader in thinking and achieving the 'impossible' to transform health and improve lives," says Bernadette Melnyk, the college's dean, who also serves as vice president for health promotion, chief wellness officer, and a professor at Ohio State. As a result, her institution is among the first of the nation's nursing colleges to teach students "to promote optimal wellbeing via telehealth and to deploy telehealth in practice," Melnyk said.

In 2016, the College of Nursing added telehealth education to clinical experiences for graduate students in the advanced nursing practice programs, and later to pre-licensure nursing courses as well. The College is also creating online, self-paced continuing education materials on telehealth for nurse practitioners (NPs) and registered nurses already in practice. In addition, the College of Nursing operates Ohio State Total Health and Wellness, a nurse practitioner-led, interprofessional, comprehensive health center that now uses telehealth to provide health care to the students, faculty, staff, and their dependents on the Lima, Ohio campus. With the assistance of registered nurses on site with patients in Lima, primary care is delivered by nurse practitioners from the Total Health and Wellness center located in Columbus, 93 miles to the southeast. These patient-provider exchanges take place through a secure, high-definition video connection over the internet.

The College plans to have its nurse practitioner students undergo preceptorships—short-term training and education with actual care practitioners—at Total Health & Wellness to learn how to conduct telehealth consultations in a team-based setting with nurses, dietitians, and pharmacists. After the initial pilot test of telehealth on the first regional campus in Lima, the college plans to deploy telehealth services at an additional regional campus beginning in 2019. The Community Health Workers (CHW) program offered by the Ohio State College of Nursing is another initiative that exemplifies "Health Care Without Walls." The community health worker program is approved by the Ohio Board of Nursing, and facilitates the educational experiences for 3 cohorts of 26 CHW students each year.

The program includes 104 classroom hours and 130 practicum hours. Classes are conducted in the evenings and on Saturdays over a 12-week period. Students in the program must have either a high school diploma or General Equivalency Diploma and pass a background check. The community health workers completing the Ohio State program are employed in various organizations in the community and are able to address population specific concerns, such as infant mortality. As a result, the community health worker program "is making an important difference in improving outcomes and the lives of underserved populations in our area," Melnyk says.

Methods to determine types and numbers of needed health workers

This report, along with companion reports from the other Health Care Without Walls work streams, recognizes that there is considerable uncertainty about what the U.S. health care delivery system will look like in 2025, and by extension, how many, and which types of existing and new workers will be needed. These uncertainties include issues related to payment, models of care, the evolving role of technology, shifts in demand and tasks for various types of workers, and how patients will respond to these changes. To begin to address how many, and which types of health care workers will be needed in the future, the Work Force Work Stream was charged with identifying methods to estimate the types and numbers of health workers that will be required to fulfill the 2025 vision.

Before exploring what methods could be used to estimate how many health care workers will be needed in the future, it is useful to understand some of the limitations of existing resources and methods that are used to project health care work force needs. The Work Force Work Stream emphasized that existing projections for these workers do not account for the evolving role of technology. For example, no projection of future physician work force needs is based on any set of assumptions about the evolving role of telehealth or telemedicine, or of artificial intelligence or enhanced forms of clinical decision support. Failure to account for how technology will affect various types of health care workers quite possibly results in an overestimation of the need for some types of workers, as well as corresponding underestimates of the need for others.

A second methodologic consideration involves ongoing difficulties in researchers' ability to effectively track the evolution of the health care work force using federally-sponsored data sources and systems. The Bureau of Labor Statistics (BLS) bases its classifications of workers—and by extension, work force projections—on the Standard Occupational Classification (SOC) system.[146] This system, which classifies workers into occupational categories as part of a national strategy to collect and disseminate data about the U.S. labor force, categorizes workers into one of 867 occupations according to their occupational definition. These occupations and related codes were revised in 2017, a process that offered an opportunity for the federal government to define new occupational codes that reflect technology-driven changes in the health care work force. However, the BLS declined to accept recommendations by the American Medical Informatics Association that would have created new codes for a variety of health informatics workers whose roles have emerged and continued to evolve in recent years.

As a result of the failure to adopt these new codes, there is no official tally of, or set of projections for, these types of workers.[147] Without detailed statistics that reflect these new types of technology- and data-driven health care jobs, it will be very challenging to determine if employers' needs are being met, if new degree programs are accommodating student volume that reflects demands of the health care labor market, and it will also be impossible to track these and related trends over time.

A third methodological consideration in health care is that past experience, including the demand for specific types of workers, is not necessarily a good predictor of what will be needed in the future. The ongoing evolution of care delivery and technology, coupled with secular trends such as new approaches to drug development, suggest that extreme caution should be exercised when using historical health care work force data to predict future demands; it is likely to be the case that using historical data to estimate future demand for specific types of health care workers will become an increasingly futile effort.

The Work Force Work Stream agreed that these methodologic issues—the need to account for the role of technology in estimating future demand for labor, the absence of SOC codes that reflect new jobs in the health care sector, and the diminishing utility of historical data in predicting future demand—create serious flaws in existing health care work force projections. The group called for development of new methods to accurately predict what types and how many health care sector jobs will be needed in the future, and that these methods should employ reliable data that reflect the realities of today's health care landscape.

However, the Work Force Work Stream also recognized the considerable difficulties associated with addressing these flawed methods, an acknowledgement that prompted the group to propose future research focusing on these challenging issues.

Other Knowledge Gaps about the Future Health Care Work Force

The Work Force Work Stream emphasized that, ideally, robust evidence must be the foundation for informed decision-making concerning the future health care work force. However, given the long pipeline for the education and training of health professionals as well as faculty and students, numerous decisions will need to be made soon despite uncertainties about the future. These decisions will involve how tomorrow's health care workers will interact with current and emerging technologies and new models of care. Although the group relied on published evidence to support the recommendations in this report, in doing so, it also highlighted gaps in the current body of research that should be filled to enable future evidence-based decision making. As noted above, some of these gaps in knowledge stem from the absence of high-quality statistics to inform on the future health care work force.

Among the research topics that can and should be pursued in the short term are studies of the impact on workers, patients, quality, and costs of the evolving models of virtual care delivery that are currently taking root in major health systems around the country. It is not too early to begin thinking about how to design and implement studies that examine work force inputs, practices, patient attitudes and outcomes, and other factors in these evolving virtual models and compare these factors to traditional models of care. As part of this process, "embedded researchers"—clinical investigators who are involved in study design and implementation as well as care delivery—could be a key source of information about qualitative issues such as how these new ways of providing care impact clinical workflow.

The Work Force Work Stream agreed that now is the time to think carefully about the most important research questions about the future health care work force and to set up high-quality studies that begin to address these questions. Ideally, this research could involve "core data collection elements" as well as flexible "modules" that could be introduced in response to changing technology or other circumstances. In this way, future research efforts could use core elements as common threads that tie long-term projects together while at the same time being able to introduce more specialized data collection modules that allows the research to examine more detailed questions without veering off course from achievement of larger objectives. Questions that could be addressed in such studies include determining what professional work force will be needed to best serve patients in the home; how informal caregivers in the home will be affected; how best to train providers in conducting virtual health care; how to staff organizations for virtual encounters; and defining the new jobs, tasks, and roles of various members of health care teams that operating in more virtual contexts.

Additional research is also needed to address the impact that various technologies are likely to have on work force supply and demand. For example, as noted above, there is growing evidence that much of the traditional work of radiologists and pathologists can be read and interpreted by machines.[132] But it is not clear how many of these professionals will be displaced completely by these technologies. Similar trends are occurring in many other physician specialty areas, and there is no doubt that technology will change demands for other types of health care workers as well. To prepare for America's future health care environment, research is needed to understand how different types of workers will be affected by ongoing technological and system-level changes.

One place to begin could be research that explores what has occurred in other industries with respect to shifts in occupational classifications due to automation, and drawing inferences that might be applicable to health care. The Work Force Work Stream agreed that the pressing need for answers to these and related questions suggests that research and other academic work should be directed to modeling the future health care work force, or at least to identifying the range of uncertainties behind existing projections.

Additional Recommendations To Support Work Force for "Health Care Without Walls" in 2025

Among the charges to the Work Force Work Stream was the task of drafting recommendations to other stakeholders, beyond those in charge of education and training of health care professionals and other workers, concerning how to ensure that America's health care work force of the future is prepared to meet the 2025 vision. The recommendations cited below are aimed chiefly at two groups: federal and state policy makers, and leaders of major health systems and their payer/partners who are developing new care delivery models.

Although these recommendations are necessarily broad and purposefully targeted at these two stakeholder groups, there was agreement among Work Force Work Stream members that these stakeholders should act immediately to begin what will undoubtedly be long-term, multi-step processes to achieve these recommendations. From a practical point of view, the work stream believes that all stakeholders have the capacity to "go after low hanging fruit" in the short term while more complex issues are worked out that will allow these groups to tackle bigger issues over the longer term.

Recommendations for federal and state policy makers

1. <u>Establish and harmonize licensure compacts</u>

    States should be encouraged or incentivized to join physician, nurse, and other health professions licensure compacts to facilitate multistate licensure and to facilitate interstate provision of care. The federal government could take on more prominent role in this process by offering incentives to states to join these compacts by a certain date, and by imposing penalties if states did not do so. A key operational aspect of this process would involve harmonization of licensure requirements for these compacts. For example, the existing physician licensure compact speeds up the process through which a physician licensed in one state can obtain a license in another state, but it still retains the separate state licensing with differing requirements from one state to another.

    Concurrently, the federal government could also begin developing and implementing a parallel process aimed at creating a national licensure construct. This construct would not preempt state licensure; it would be an alternate process that states could opt into voluntarily if desired. Over time, if national licensure proved attractive to clinicians and the multistate systems that often hire them, states might harmonize their requirements with the national licensure process, or drop their separate state licensure systems altogether. Among the benefits of such a strategy would be the forging of a national market in the health care work force, with the ability of health care workers to work across state lines, a basic element of virtual health care delivery.

2. Expand scope of practice

There is a need to develop and enact model legislation on scope of practice that aims to facilitate health care providers' ability to practice at the top of their licenses. There is considerable untapped potential in the existing health care work force—particularly among nursing assistants, community health workers, and pharmacists. The unutilized potential in these labor pools can be accessed with new regulations that allow properly trained and certified professionals to deliver higher levels of care. Such legislation would help move the country toward the 2025 vision of a health care system that is heavily focused on primary care, and in which this care can be provided in venues that are most convenient for patients and their families.

One example of model legislation already in existence is the Model Act[148] created by the National Council of State Boards of Nursing, which sets forth provisions for optimal scope of practice for various categories of nurses, including advanced practice nurses. Comparable model statutes should be created for other types of providers as described above.

Recommendations for health systems and payers

1. Treat the whole person

The Work Force Work Stream encourages a shift in resources toward distributed supports that address both physical health and supportive services that influence health like housing, transportation, and food. Efforts to recognize and address the reality that non-clinical factors impact health will result in more effective and cost-effective health and care.

2. Re-imagine primary care delivery

New technologies and ways of providing primary health care are available now, and bringing these into primary care, and creating the capabilities in the work force to use them, constitutes the obvious first place to begin creating a "Health Care Without Walls" system. Health care organizations, together with payers, should recognize the great value of these existing resources and move aggressively to optimize them by supporting development of diverse teams of workers, each of whom works at the top of license.

The Work Force to Support Health Care Without Walls: Chapter 4 in Brief

1. NEHI's vision for health care in 2025 is that health care will increasingly be accessed and delivered "without walls." Patients will receive more care than they do now in their homes, schools, and other community-based venues and "distributed" settings out of conventional health care settings, such as hospitals and physicians' offices. It will be possible to provide many forms of health care across state, regional, and even national borders. Vast amounts of data will be turned into actionable information to assist clinical decision-making; care will be delivered far more often than at present by multidisciplinary teams of providers, whose clinical competencies will be accompanied by new skill sets that facilitate application of technology and informatics in routine patient care; and these multidisciplinary teams will also address the social and economic determinants of health that often drive illness and care needs.

2. All of these changes will have a profound impact on the health care work force—the people who will be delivering care to patients in these ways. As these more distributed forms of health care evolve, the roles of almost all types of health care professionals are likely to change substantially, and it will be critical to have the health care work force be as flexible and adaptable as possible to accommodate the changes. New capabilities and practices will have to be created to provide excellent health care in more distributed settings; more types of workers, such as community health workers, may be needed, and the tasks performed by current types of workers, in terms of what they do and how they do it, will change.

3. A health care work force that fully utilized technology could markedly increase access to care, especially in underserved areas. However, because labor represents such a large cost component of health care, keeping that care affordable will demand making the most efficient use possible of labor through increased productivity, not simply having more bodies equipped with more technology to provide it. Advancing technology may provide

opportunities both to supplant some types of labor, as well as to augment the decision-making skills of health professionals to such a degree that "task shifting" of labor from higher-skilled to less-skilled workers may also become a reality. To make such task shifting possible, it will be increasingly important to have all health professionals, and particularly non-physician health care professionals, trained, certified, and empowered to practice at the top of their licenses.

4. The Work Force work stream of the Health Care Without Walls Initiative articulated a vision for a qualified work force capable of meeting the health and health care needs of Americans, and that advances the health of Americans, not just the care. It sought to describe what types of education and training would prepare the future work force to provide safe, efficacious, efficient, accessible, cost-effective, and culturally appropriate care in distributed settings. It also considered ways to increase the rewarding aspects of working in the health care sector and minimizing frustration and burnout.

5. The Work Force work stream reviewed many different projections of the types of health care workers that will be needed in the future, and found that none of them incorporated any assumptions about how increased use of various technologies would affect either the supply of or demand for such workers. As noted throughout this report, advances in technology, changes in scope of practice, and expanded application of artificial intelligence and other information technologies into the health care sector will undoubtedly result in reduced work force needs in some fields or occupations, and increased demand in others. Because most existing projections do not take such factors into account, they are deeply flawed, and don't serve as a useful guide to planning for the future work force. New methodologies should be developed that begin to take various assumptions about the use of technologies, such as artificial intelligence, into account.

6. To ensure the greatest productivity, flexibility, and adaptability of labor in the health care sector, and to make the best use of the nation's investment in training health care professionals, substantial changes are needed in licensure. regulation. As set forth in the Regulatory chapter of this volume, states should be encouraged or incentivized to join physician, nurse, and other health professions licensure compacts to facilitate multistate licensure to facilitate interstate provision of care. The federal government should take on a more prominent role in this process by offering incentives to states to

join these compacts by a certain date, and by imposing penalties if states do not do so. Concurrently, the federal government could also begin developing and implementing a parallel process aimed at creating a national licensure construct that states could opt into voluntarily if desired. There is also a need to develop and enact model legislation within states on scope of practice that aims to facilitate health care providers' ability to practice at the top of their licenses.

7. Although the current health care work force contains a talented pool of workers with tremendous potential to meet the needs of a more technology-enabled, distributed health care system, many of these workers do not have adequate training and skills for this purpose. Many changes will thus need to occur in education and training of health care workers. What's more, given the long pipeline for the education and training of health professionals as well as faculty and students, numerous decisions will need to be made soon despite uncertainties about the future.

8. The federal government, states, and institutions and organizations involved in higher education and training of health professionals should define new competencies that some or all types of health care workers should have in the future to deliver more virtual care. They should also attempt to define new categories of workers who will be needed, or to define how existing categories of workers should evolve to meet a changing health care environment.

9. Institutions and organizations will need to overhaul existing degree-granting programs to reflect advances in technology and new models of care. They will need to increase integration of technology and informatics into curricula, and improve how the use of technology is taught, with a focus on setting targets for the development of skills and competencies appropriate for different types of health professionals. Degree-granting programs must provide workers with instruction in areas such as health informatics, virtual health care, team-based care, and working in collaboration with community-based organizations. They will need to create new certification and degree programs for new types of health care workers, such as community health workers or virtual specialists and technicians. Institutions and organizations also should increase their emphasis on inter-professional education that teaches team-based care.

10. Faculty members at many institutions that provide higher education of health professionals are often far removed from clinical practice. These institutions, and their umbrella organizations, will need to provide opportunities for faculty development in technology use and instruction within teaching institutions.

11. Institutions and organizations will need to provide more practical opportunities for continuing education for health care professionals, to allow them to obtain the necessary skills to deliver more virtual, team-based care, and to function effectively in a rapidly-changing health care environment. Expanded online continuing education should be a priority. Institutions and organizations also should emphasize "stackable" credentials in virtual care delivery: e.g., certificates that can be obtained for training to be added on top of an existing degree.

12. Robust evidence should be the foundation for informed decision-making concerning the future health care work force, but there are multiple gaps in the current body of research. The federal and state governments, as well as private institutions, should fund the design and implementation of studies to examine work force inputs, practices, patient attitudes and outcomes, and other factors in evolving virtual models, and to compare these factors to traditional models of care. Research is also needed to understand how different types of workers will be affected by ongoing technological and system-level changes, with findings ultimately incorporated into more meaningful work force projections.

◆ ◆ ◆

End Notes, Chapter 4

[124] "Task Shifting: Global Recommendations and Guidelines," The World Health Organization, accessed April 3, 2018, http://www.who.int/healthsystems/TTR-TaskShifting.pdf?ua=1.

[125] Clemens Scott Kruse, et al., "Barriers to Electronic Health Record Adoption: a Systematic Literature Reviews," *Journal of Medical Systems* 40, no. 12(October 2016):252, DOI: 10.1007/s10916-016-0628-9.

[126] "Improving Access to Care," Campaign for Action, accessed January 14, 2018, https://campaignforaction.org/issue/improving-access-to-care/.

[127] Mary Ann Kliethermes, "Understanding health care billing basics," *Pharmacy Today* 23, no 7(2017):57-68, https://www.pharmacytoday.org/article/S1042-0991(17)30973-8/fulltext.

[128] Samantha Artiga and Elizabeth Hinton, "Beyond Health Care: The Role of Social Determinants in Promoting Health and Health Equity," Kaiser Family Foundation, accessed December 7, 2017, https://www.kff.org/disparities-policy/issue-brief/beyond-health-care-the-role-of-social-determinants-in-promoting-health-and-health-equity/.

[129] See https://www.medicaid.gov/medicaid/ltss/downloads/ltss-expenditures-2014.pdf.

[130] See https://www.managedcaremag.com/archives/2018/4/3-social-determinants-strategies.

[131] "AMIA Accreditation Committee," AMIA, accessed January 16, 2018, https://www.amia.org/sites/default/files/AMIA-Health-Informatics-Core-Competencies-for-CAHIIM.PDF.

[132] Saurabh Jha and Eric Topol, "Adapting to Artificial Intelligence: Radiologists and Pathologists as Information Specialists," *JAMA* 316, no. 22, (December 13, 2016): 2353-2354, DOI: 10.1001/jama.2016.17438.

[133] Mark A. Munger, David N. Sundwall, and Michael Feehan, "Integrating family medicine and community pharmacy to improve patient access to quality primary care and enhance health outcomes," *American Journal of Pharmaceutical Education* 82, no.4(2018):6572, https://doi.org/10.5688/ajpe6572.

[134] "First global conference on task shifting," World Health Organization, accessed March 19, 2018, http://www.who.int/mediacentre/events/meetings/task_shifting/en/.

[135] "Task shifting: global recommendations and guidelines," World Health Organization, accessed March 19, 2018, http://www.who.int/workforcealliance/knowledge/resources/taskshifting_guidelines/en/.

[136] Esther Hing and Chun-Ju Hsiao, "State Variability in Supply of Office-based Primary Care Providers: United States, 2012," NCHS Data Brief, no. 151, *Hyattsville, MD: National Center for Health Statistics* (2014).

[137] Jonathan Peterson, "Where Are the Doctors You'll Need?," AARP, April 2016, https://www.aarp.org/health/conditions-treatments/info-2016/geriatrician-geriatric-doctor-physician.html.

[138] Michael Nochomovitz and Rahul Sharma, "Is It Time for a New Medical Specialty?," *JAMA* 319, no.5 (February 6, 2018):437-438, doi:10.1001/jama.2017.17094.

[139] Ibid.

[140] Mutaz Shegewi, "Implementing Robots in Healthcare," Robotics Tomorrow, August, 31, 2017,https://www.roboticstomorrow.com/article/2017/08/implementing-robots-in-healthcare/10538.

[141] Mutaz Shegewi, "IDC Survey: Provider Investment Plans for Robotics," IDC, June 2017, https://www.idc.com/getdoc.jsp?containerId=US42725617.

[142] Dean Arnold and Tim Wilson, "What doctor? Why AI and robotics will define New Health," PWC, accessed December 13, 2017, https://www.pwc.com/gx/en/industries/healthcare/publications/ai-robotics-new-health.html.

[143] See, for example, Shreya Kangovi et al., " Community Health Worker Support for Disadvantaged Patients With Multiple Chronic Diseases: A Randomized Clinical Trial," *American Journal of Public Health* 107, no. 10(2017):1660-1667, DOI:10.2105/AJPH.2017.303985.

[144] See, for example, Jonathan D. Campbell et al., "Community Health Worker Home Visits for Medicaid-Enrolled Children With Asthma: Effects on Asthma Outcomes and Costs," *American Journal of Public Health* 105, no. 11(November 2015):2366-72, DOI: 10.2105/AJPH.2015.302685.

[145] See, for example, https://www.healthconnectone.org/nachw-progress-and-purpose/.

[146] "Standard Occupational Classification- Revision for 2010," Office of the Federal Register, accessed January 17, 2018, https://www.federalregister.gov/documents/2006/05/16/E6-7415/standard-occupational-classification-revision-for-2010.

[147] "Standard Occupational Classification (SOC)- Revision for 2018; Notice," Office of the Federal Register, accessed January 17, 2018, https://www.federalregister.gov/documents/2014/05/22/2014-11913/standard-occupational-classification-soc-revision-for-2018-notice.

[148] See https://ncsbn.org/14_Model_Act_0914.pdf.

SCENARIO 7: A PREGNANT WOMAN AT HIGH RISK FOR PREGNANCY COMPLICATIONS AND PREMATURE BIRTH

AMANDA IS A woman of color in her early 30s and in the first trimester of pregnancy—her first. She works at a low-wage job and, given her uncertain hours, has difficulty getting to prenatal appointments at the federally qualified health center where she receives care. She is overweight, but she gave up smoking when she became pregnant, and she now wants to do her best to have a healthy baby.

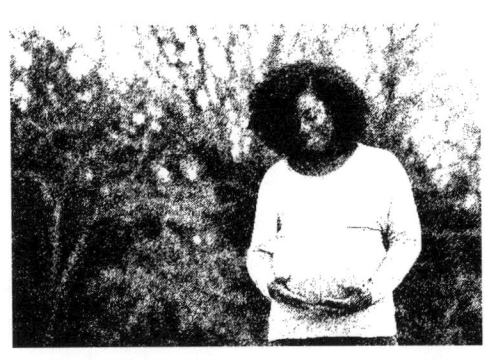

Amanda's care team at the health center is very supportive, and at the same time, very concerned. Poor health before pregnancy, along with inadequate access to prenatal care, may contribute to pregnancy-related complications such as gestational diabetes and preeclampsia. Both pregnancy-related death rates, and postpartum maternal death rates, are on the rise in the United States. Babies born to women of color in the United States can face a 130 percent higher infant death rate than babies born to white women.

Another concern is pre-term birth—birth before 37 weeks of gestation. Giving birth pre-term can happen to any pregnant woman, and affects nearly 1 in every 10 infants born in the country. There are also substantial racial and ethnic disparities in rates of prematurity in the United States, with African American women and infants experiencing about a 50 percent higher pre-term birth rate than white women. In 2007, the Institute of Medicine (now the National Academy of Medicine) reported that the costs associated with premature birth in the United States were $26.2 billion each year, including $16.9 billion in medical and health care costs for babies and $1.9 billion in labor and delivery expenses for mothers. Without appropriate treatment, survivors of complications of pre-term birth are at increased risk of lifelong disability and poor quality of life.

Fortunately, the health center is participating in a federally-funded program to test innovative ways to improve maternity care for mothers on Medicaid (a program that now pays for nearly half the births annually in the nation). The center will be paid under a new "bundle" formula to coordinate the care of eligible pregnant women, and to link with other organizations along a care continuum, including local hospitals and birthing centers. The bundled payment gives the center the ability to experiment with new ways of caring for pregnant women—some of which involve new technology, but others of which involve care providers and care modalities that haven't been widely employed in U.S. maternity care until recently.

On her first visit to the health center following a positive pregnancy test, Amanda meets with her care coordinator, who explains how Amanda will be cared for during her pregnancy. She will have an initial meeting at the center with an obstetrician-gynecologist, during which she'll also meet other members of her care team, including a nurse practitioner and a doula—a trained assistant who offers emotional and physical support to a woman before, during, and after childbirth. The doula will be her most regular point of contact, and will interact with Amanda on almost a daily basis. At least once a month, Amanda will come to the health center to see the ob/gyn and consult with the nurse practitioner and a nutritionist. In what is known as the "centering" model, she will also have a group visits with other pregnant women, typically in the evenings after work, to receive education and obtain peer support. If she can't make it to the group visit in person, she can also join via Skype or FaceTime.

On the technology front, Amanda receives a new smart phone, on which she'll receive text messages from her doula, as well as an artificial-intelligence-enabled app that she can use to consult about any medical issues. She is also given a digitally-connected blood pressure cuff for remote monitoring of signs of preeclampsia, or high blood pressure during pregnancy, as well as a handheld ultrasound device. The nurse practitioner shows her how to use these two devices regularly to transmit her blood pressure readings, and ultrasound images of her baby, to the health center. The health center staff also helps Amanda install apps for Uber and Lyft so she can use these services at no out-of-pocket cost to get to her health care appointments. Over Amanda's phone, the nurse practitioner and doula send her links to videos so that she can learn more about how the baby is developing; how to prepare for delivery; and options for delivering her baby in a hospital, or in a birthing center with a midwife.

Amanda's pregnancy goes well through her second trimester, and she is in the early stages of the third trimester when the remote monitoring device detects elevated blood pressure, a possible sign of preeclampsia. Her ob/gyn prescribes an antihypertensive medication and a corticosteroid, which ease the problem. Amanda meets other pregnant women at the "centering" group meetings who have also developed preeclampsia during their current or previous pregnancies. They share their concerns about their own health, and that of their babies, and also coping strategies, and agree to call each other in between centering meetings to provide moral support.

As Amanda approaches her delivery date, she watches a shared decision-making video that explains various delivery options, including normal vaginal birth with and without anesthesia, and elective and emergency cesarean sections. She learns about the potential dangers of elective C-sections, as well as elective pre-term inductions. The more she learns, the more she is increasingly persuaded that she'll opt for a normal vaginal birth without anesthesia. She is also increasingly drawn to the notion of giving birth in a birthing center with a certified nurse-midwife.

In a telehealth consultation with the midwife, and the rest of Amanda's care team, she is walked through the options. She learns that, even if she elects the midwifery option, her ob/gyn will remain on call in case any emergencies arise. She also learns about the quick hand-offs that are possible from the birthing center to the local hospital in the event that she needs an emergency c-section. Several days before her due date, contractions begin, and she calls her doula, who comes immediately. After timing the contractions for a couple of hours, they leave for the birthing center, where the midwife is waiting.

Several hours go by, during which Amanda labors for a while in a bathtub, walks around the floor, and eventually asks for and receives a "walking epidural" shot that dulls the pain. The doula gives her regular massages to help her relax. Eventually, after 7 hours of labor, an overjoyed Amanda gives birth to a healthy 9-pound baby boy. She names him Christian.

After a few hours of sleep, Amanda meets with a lactation consultant, and a pediatrician comes by to check on Christian. Then, Amanda, the baby, and the doula head to Amanda's home. The doula will stay with her for the next several days to help Amanda begin breastfeeding, and instruct her further in caring for the baby. The nurse practitioner comes by daily for the first few days for visits, and then checks in regularly by telehealth thereafter.

Amanda's care team at the health center is well aware of the fact that many mothers experience post-partum depression, and that the majority of maternal deaths take place during the first year post delivery, rather than at the time of delivery. As a result, a psychiatric social worker is added to the care team to have regular consultations with Amanda and the doula. When Amanda feels tired or blue, the social worker provides support, and also urges Amanda to contact other mothers from the "centering" group for peer support. Amanda's care coordinator also visits to talk through Amanda's return to work after her brief maternity leave, and options for child care services for Christian.

As a single mother, Amanda has a long road ahead to provide for herself and her son. But looking at her baby, she can't believe her good fortune—and can't say enough good things about the care team that brought her and Christian to this happy point in life.

♦ ♦ ♦

CHAPTER 5:
HUMAN FACTORS IN DESIGNING HEATH CARE WITHOUT WALLS

A S PREVIOUS CHAPTERS in this volume have described, the Health Care Without Walls vision for 2025 is predicated on the fact that profound changes are occurring in how health care services and supports are delivered, with care moving out of conventional health care settings thanks to technologies such as telehealth and remote monitoring. Many of these technologies will widely be used outside of the "walls" of the health care system, as patients receive monitoring, advice, and care, and conduct their own self-care, in settings including worksites, schools, their own homes.

These more distributed forms of care delivery, coupled with a greater emphasis on meeting the social needs of individuals in their homes and communities, will cause further sweeping changes in the ways that individuals and health care professionals engage with each other—not just for given care episodes, but over their lifetimes. These changes will affect how individuals and their care providers interact with each other, and with technology.

Consideration of these changes thus require a focus on human factors— defined as "the scientific discipline concerned with the understanding of interactions among humans and other elements of a system."[149] The field of human factors, as a result, is "concerned with applying what is known about human behavior, abilities, limitations, and other characteristics to the design of systems, tasks/activities, environments, and equipment/technologies."[150] As more virtual encounters replace the traditional in-person visit, for example, how will individuals respond differently to their health care providers? What will happen when patients interact with non-human interfaces, such as avatars? Why might people react differently to a robot that features a human-like face versus one that resembles a mere machine?

The Human Factors Work Stream of NEHI's Health Care Without Walls Initiative thus focused on the likely interactions that will take place between humans and technologies as the care patterns described in earlier chapters of this volume evolve. Among the types of interactions it considered were the following:

- Use of technologies, such as mobile applications or monitoring devices, by consumers and patients to support their health and manage illness;

- Use of technologies by health care professionals to deliver health and care services, such as clinical consultations delivered virtually via video, and augmented with digital biometric devices such as glucometers and otoscopes;

- Use of technologies to displace humans and actually provide care to patients—for example, by robots;

- Use of technologies to create "smart" environments that constantly sense environmental factors (e.g. air quality or the weather); combine these data with individual patient biometric data; and feed the information back into patients' electronic health records or applications.

As Health Care Without Walls unfolds, human factors will determine to what extent, and how successfully, these technologies are integrated into health care and the lives of patients. Too frequently, these human factors have been given short shrift. A 2009 article by Suzanne Buck in the *Journal of Telemedicine and Telecare*[151] described the situation as it applied then to telemedicine: "Much attention is paid to the technical aspects of telemedicine in the development of new applications, but the enthusiasm about what is technically possible very often leads to the user acceptance of such products being neglected. The number of successful and sustainable telemedicine applications would be much higher if developers concentrated more on matters related to the cognitive-emotional situation of the users involved in telemedicine."

Sharing the belief that human factors are frequently underweighted in discussions about technology in health care, the Human Factors Work Stream had six major goals, as follows:

1) Taking into account the vision developed by the Technology Work Stream as to what the delivery of health care will look like in 2025, and accompanying patient and population scenarios, define the relevant human factors issues that should be considered as new care models develop.

2) Examine human factors behind interventions to improve the *health* of Americans, not just those designed to deliver health care.

3) Identify the core human factors issues that technology developers, health systems, educational and training systems and others should address in order to facilitate the evolution of a patient-centric, distributed health care system.

4) Recommend changes in public policy, and within health systems and other organizations, to support the 2025 Health Care Without Walls vision.

Human Factors and Health Care Technology: The Backdrop

As members of the Human Factors Work Stream repeatedly underscored, any discussion about technology and health care can never be confined only to technology. Emerging technologies must be considered as part of the broader "sociotechnical" system,[152,153] in which technologies interact with the social and physical realities of the world and with people's beliefs and abilities. Understanding the sociotechnical system requires a multidisciplinary view, using approaches including human factors and ergonomics, behavioral economics, sociology, psychology, and human-centered design. Exploring new technologies through this broad, multidisciplinary perspective is essential in order to fully understand the promises and pitfalls of a new world of "Health Care Without Walls."

To understand the sociotechnical system, one must consider how people within the system will interact with and respond to the technologies, and to the entire notion of distributed care, asking questions such as the following:

- How will users respond to technology? What do we know about how users respond differently to virtual versus physical interactions?

- How will human biases, beliefs, and preferences influence how technologies will be created; whether technologies will be adopted; and how they will be implemented and used?

- What generational, ethnic, cultural, and/or racial differences influence how people respond to technology?

- Will the use of more technologies in health care disparately affect people depending on their socioeconomic status or other factors?

- Will people with different abilities and levels of literacy be included or left behind as systems evolve?

- Will the influence of social determinants on health be exacerbated or mitigated with technology, or with movement of care to more distributed settings?

- How will the roles of patients and providers change around the use of technologies that virtualize health and care services?

- How can health care systems employing new technologies be designed in ways that will benefit all users? What design principles should be employed?

- How do we make technologies so easy to use that patients and providers will readily adopt them?

- How do we use technology to minimize error and risk in all facets of the healthcare system?

- Can technology be a barrier to better communication between patients and providers? If so, how can these barriers be overcome?

- When do technologies create better communications and interactions than those that take place without them? When are these communications and interactions worse with technologies present?

- Since people are likely to adopt technology at different stages—early adopters, for example, versus later ones—how can health systems and others plan effectively for graduated introduction of technologies? What are the implications for those who might never adopt technologies?

- How should technology be designed to be efficiently and safely used in various physical environments (e.g., under low lighting conditions)? How should the physical environment be adapted and redesigned to facilitate use of technology (e.g., adequate physical ergonomics of workstations)?

Understanding the sociotechnical system surrounding use of a technology means answering these and other questions. It also means exploring the appropriate balance between technology and humans, and the impact that technology may have on human relationships. Will technologies overcome barriers to human-to-human communication and connection, or create new ones? Will technologies exacerbate social isolation and loneliness, which are dangerous to health?

Will technologies be easy for people of all physical abilities to use? Will they be useful in a range of physical settings, for example, in both workplaces and homes? Will patients and providers be able to choose the technologies with which they are comfortable, or will there be a one-size-fits-all approach? Will the health care work force be able to use technologies effectively, and how must it be educated or trained to do so? Will the integration of more technologies into health care have implications not just for health and health care, but also for society as a whole?

Finally, the potential impact of emerging technologies should be evaluated from the perspective that the ultimate goal is not simply to improve the delivery of health *care*, but rather to ensure optimal health—physical, mental, and social—for all individuals throughout their lives. Technologies should not just be employed to "deliver" care, but to support individuals' health and self-care, encourage healthy behavior change, and foster community support networks to reinforce health. The work stream participants stressed the urgency of making sure that moving toward a more distributed care system constitutes a step forward in addressing these goals, rather than potentially doing an even worse job in achieving total health than the current health care system.

The work stream also prioritized a list of features that technologies used in a more distributed system of health care should incorporate, as follows:

- **Human-centered design**: Humans have a range of physical, mental, and emotional needs, desires, and limits that influence how well they function in any setting. The field of human-centered design has evolved to take these factors into account, and it should be employed in constructing new models of technology-enabled virtual care. As described by Ideo, a leading human-centered design firm, "Human-centered design is a creative approach to problem solving... It's a process that starts with the people you're designing for and ends with new solutions that are tailor made to suit their needs. Human-centered design is all about building a deep empathy with the people you're designing for; generating tons of ideas; building a bunch of prototypes; sharing what you've made with the people you're designing for; and eventually putting your innovative new solution out in the world."[154] True human-centered design also requires validating through observation and study that any solutions generated actually work for human beings in the "real world," not just in a laboratory or other idealized setting.

- **Ease of use**. Technologies should be easy to use and "frictionless" for users, seamlessly integrated into their lives so that it becomes an almost invisible part of the health care journey. Technologies should be viewed as the engine under the hood of the car—essential, but largely out of sight.

- **Interoperability.** A necessary element of frictionless and seamless health care experience is the ability of systems and devices to exchange data; to allow data to follow the patient; and to present data in such a way that they are clearly understood and actionable for users.

- **Integration and convergence of all components.** Technologies should enable care in a way that all components are seamlessly connected. For example, a patient at home should be able to use an online app to summon a provider to the home; the visiting provider to use a point-of-care diagnostic or an ultrasound device; and the data from these activities should be able to be uploaded directly into an electronic health record (EHR) or other repository of patient data.

- **Safety:** Technologies should not only be safe when used correctly, but should incorporate fail-safe mechanisms and backstops that will prevent injury or death in the event that they are not used correctly.

The work stream also emphasized the need to strike an appropriate balance between human and technological intervention; the potential for technology to hinder or help the coordination of care; and the need to plan for an abundance of data generated by technology and the human capacity to absorb and process it. The following sections describe these general issues, and then turn to the specific issues that will affect different patients and providers.

General Issues

Appropriate Balance Between Humans and Technology

There are widespread and deeply rooted beliefs and biases about the appropriate use of technology, particularly regarding the use of technology in health care. These beliefs lead to assumptions that certain types of care are better, and preferences for these types of care—for example, in-person care as opposed to virtual care. However, a growing body of research shows that these preferences are not always supported by real-world experiences and research.

For example, a widely-held belief is that interactions between humans are preferable to interactions with technology. However, sometimes technology has benefits that outweigh the presumed benefits of human-to-human interaction. For example, research by Timothy Bickmore and others has found that people of all ages often will share more complete, accurate, and honest information with a virtual "person" than they do with human clinicians.[155] Other research has shown that patients are more open to coaching and are more compliant with care plans when they come from a virtual provider.[156]

For example, a study in the United Kingdom found that people with depression responded well to therapy that was delivered in conjunction with virtual reality and avatars. Patients wore a virtual reality headset that projected life-sized images of an adult and a child; by identifying with and speaking to the avatars, the patients in effect became engaged in a process of delivering therapy to themselves. with therapy.[157]

The advantages of such virtual providers, or of providing care in virtual environments, may be due in part to the fact that these interactions can be tailored to the preferences of patients. In some virtual systems, patients can create provider-avatars that are the same race, age and gender as they are. There is less of a hierarchical relationship between a patient and a virtual provider, compared with the more common patient-physician interaction. For these reasons, it is possible that patients who may be reluctant to tell their actual care providers about certain delicate issues, such as the fact that they are struggling to comply with care plans, may be more likely to share this information with a virtual provider.

Another widely held belief is that in-person care is best, compared to care provided via phone, email, video, or other technologies. However, this belief may be diminishing as more people become familiar with eVisits, or clinical encounters that take place via secure messaging systems, as well as with other forms of telehealth and telemedicine, and recognize that these remote interactions can improve their access to health care providers with little to no detriment to care. Care delivered with the aid of technologies such as virtual reality can also be more "immersive" than traditional in-person care alone. For example, virtual reality is being used in some long-term care settings "to help residents with cognitive impairment and dementia unlock memories and stimulate emotions and interaction." [158]

Another example of a well-received use of technology from overseas is "Florence," or "Flo," named for the renowned nursing leader Florence Nightingale and used in England's National Health Service. As described by the NHS, Florence is primarily a text messaging service that links patients' mobile phones to clinicians' computer systems and can be used in almost any health care setting—and "for any condition where the patient at home might benefit from motivation and prompting; questions or education; or reporting symptoms and home measurements such as blood pressure, weight, oxygen saturation etc."[159] " Patients receive text messages that are devised by clinicians, but that appear to come from the friendly and chatty "Flo." Patients report that Flo "behaves like a real person" and that their level of engagement rises accordingly.[160] The system is now being replicated in the United States, where the Veterans Health Administration has begun using a similar text-messaging system with patients known as "Annie."

Elsewhere in the United States, many patients are already familiar with telemedicine applications such as emailing a provider with a question or conducting a visit over video chat. Other applications extend telemedicine even further; for example, some neonatal intensive care units, such as the one at Memorial Hermann Memorial City Medical Center in Houston, allow families to observe their infants remotely by livestreamed video, and to obtain information about their weight gain, sleep patterns, or other issues remotely.[161,162] This technology has served as a way for families to feel more connected to their infants even though they cannot always be present in the NICU. Although families still need person-to-person connection with their infants' care providers, these connections can also be facilitated by technology—such as video conferencing—if circumstances require.

In addition to these uses of technology to provide virtual or remote care, technology can also be used to facilitate non-traditional care, such as peer-to-peer support. For example, Big White Wall is a social peer support platform in the United

Kingdom for people with mental health issues.¹⁶³ Although individuals can book appointments with actual clinical providers through the site, they can also engage in peer support exchanges with similarly disposed individuals, such as people suffering from depression. These exchanges are monitored by a clinical provider, who can step in to contact a given individual if needed, but the provider does not actually facilitate or participate in the group. The platform enables patients to provide emotional support to their peers, while reducing the burden on health care providers.

Other organizations have developed online platforms to deliver mental and behavioral health support in tandem with health systems, payers, and others. SilverCloud Health Limited is a global provider of evidence-based online programs addressing conditions such as depression, anxiety and stress, as well as long-term chronic conditions such as diabetes, chronic obstructive pulmonary disease, and cardiovascular disease). More than 200 health systems, insurers, and academic institutions now use SilverCloud's onlineplatform; as of 2018, for example, 26 U.S. universities offer the platform for students and staff.¹⁶⁴ Another company, Lantern, offers mobile-based cognitive behavioral therapy to help patients deal with such issues as stress, anxiety, and body image.¹⁶⁵ It also partners with employers and health care providers to make the service available to workers and patients, who work virtually with a human coach and through a mobile app in 10-minute sessions.

Since the need for mental and behavioral health services in particular will probably always exceed the capacity of the mental health work force, enabling more of this type of peer support or supported self-care through technology is likely to be an important avenue for addressing mental health needs. Digital support systems can also increase and extend mental health and other clinical providers' range. For example, clinicians can remotely train, supervise, and assist community health workers and other peer counselors in the field, even offering them real-time decision support as needed.

As these types of technologies and approaches become more widespread, and patients and providers become more comfortable and see the benefits, the automatic preference for human-to-human interaction and in-person care is likely to fade. These preferences may to some degree be generational, in that younger individuals, who have grown up interacting with and relying on a wide variety of technologies, may be more comfortable with or even prefer virtual interactions over in-person ones.

A recent survey for the Employee Benefit Research Institute illustrates the point. The survey compared attitudes toward health care among millennials (the demographic cohort with birth years ranging from 1977 to 2000) with those of

Generation X (those born 1966-1976) and with Baby Boomers (1945-65). Millennials were less likely than earlier generations to have a primary care provider; to believe that it was important that their primary care provider knew them and their medical history personally; and that their primary care provider was aware of all of the other medical care that they receive. They were also less likely to say that they were comfortable telling their primary care provider about their health issues.[166]

On the other hand, even members of the millennial generation and younger are probably likely to value the convenience and efficiency of online care at some points, but also want more person-to-person interactions at others. For example, in consulting with care providers in the case of very serious illness. Ultimately, health care in the future and without walls will become the full range of health and care services provided with a mix of technology-enabled self-care, virtual clinical services, and in-person services in combination—the best of both in-person and virtual.

As a result, whatever the potential benefits of virtual and remote care, the patient-provider relationship will remain important, and will still require core capacities of listening, connection, and trust. Time will still need to be built into all forms of clinical encounters for patients and providers to connect and build relationships. Clinicians will still need to be trained to create rich interactions and relationships even if they are delivering care over video platforms and with other technologies. An appropriate balance and integration must be struck between the roles of technology and human beings. The art will be in determining the best use of technologies and humans, and deploying each at the proper points in the health care system.

Care Coordination in Health Care

A longstanding issue in health care has been the adequacy—or absence—of care coordination, defined as "a set of practitioner behaviors and information systems intended to bring together health services, patient needs, and streams of information to facilitate the delivery of care." The goal of this coordination is to meet the six aims of quality care set forth in the Institute of Medicine's 2001 report, Crossing the Quality Chasm: care should be safe, effective, efficient, equitable, patient-centered, and timely.[167] It is generally agreed that care coordination, although having improved in some respects in recent years, is still insufficient, and often woefully so. The Human Factors Work Stream spent some time considering the impact of greater use of technologies in care coordination, both positive and negative.

On the negative side, there is admittedly some risk that greater use of technology and virtual care could make care coordination even worse – for example, by exacerbating such issues as handoffs and transitions from one provider to another. For example, technology could enable a patient to receive remote care from multiple providers in different places, but these providers might not have the infrastructure in place to communicate effectively with one another. Without a care navigator or coordinator, critical information could be lost—or large volumes of data and information that are collected could go un-analyzed and not acted upon. Treatment plans devised by different providers caring for a given patient could be inconsistent or incompatible with each other. Handoffs between providers could be problematic, and patients could slip between the cracks.

On the positive side, technology can also be used to enhance care coordination, through such avenues as real-time remote monitoring of patients' health status, and various decision-support tools to assist patients and providers in making treatment decisions. Health information technologies such as electronic health record systems can also help identify different providers who are the de facto members of a patient's care team, even if they are not organized as a formal care team; can link these separate providers to coordinate care; can involve them in such processes as shared decision making with patients, or obtaining second opinions; and can feed back to them information obtained by remote monitoring of patients symptoms or test results. [168]

Technology also could be harnessed to address specific existing and potential care coordination challenges. For example, avatars backed by artificial or augmented intelligence could be employed as coaches or patient navigators to provide coordination services at a reasonable cost.[169] A rough analogue that already exists in the non-health care field is uAspire[170], a program that provides coaching to students and their families about financing college and university educations. The program is paid for through a variety of sources, including government grants, colleges and universities, and high schools. A health care navigator avatar could be created along these lines to serve as a consistent and knowledgeable source of counsel to patients, ensuring that patients are informed and involved in decisions about their care, including about financial issues. Text-based sources of support, such as Text4Baby[171], which offers tips and advice to pregnant women and mothers of children up to age 12 months, could be built out with avatars, artificial intelligence, and additional capabilities to increase the level of personalized support for individuals.

Issues in Processing and Using Data and Information

As noted in earlier chapters in this volume, future health technologies—particularly those that allow patients to regularly collect biometric data in their homes—will generate nearly unfathomable amounts of data.[172] Already existing technologies, such as wearable monitors, result in large amounts of data, and physicians express widely varying views about whether they have any need or responsibility to evaluate it. As the volume and complexity of data collected grows, it is unclear who or what will store, monitor, analyze, and act upon this information.

For example, for patients with diabetes, versions now exist of an "artificial pancreas," which monitors patients' glucose levels around the clock with the aid of glucometers built into patches worn on the skin that are linked directly to wearable insulin pumps. Such systems have positively transformed the profoundly complex task of managing diabetes to allow real-time, precise adjustments of patients' insulin levels. However, issues have also arisen in that patients are not always able to see the data that their devices generate, or alter or control the settings and underlying algorithms that govern the process of adjusting and delivering insulin through the pumps. As a result, the Open Artificial Pancreas System project (https://openaps.org) has formed as a grassroots effort to assist people in "hacking" these systems to give patients the control they desire.

Such systems as the artificial pancreas raise key questions: How can large volumes of data be presented in a usable and useful manner for action, decision-making and/or monitoring? Or, as addressed in the regulatory chapter of this volume, how can algorithms that govern many of these technologies be made more transparent for patients? In-home monitoring technologies such as weight scales or blood pressure cuffs will produce data at least daily, and these data need to be monitored to identify trends. Patients may have multiple providers and several remote monitoring systems, and unless they are affiliated with a particular integrated or organized delivery system, it is not clear who or what would pay attention to the data produced and act as the lead monitor, decision-maker, or actor who takes the next steps in delivering care.

The field of cognitive psychology, and a growing body of evidence around such issues as "information overload,"[173] "alert fatigue,"[174] and the brain's difficulties with multi-tasking,[175,176] illuminate the challenges that people have in processing large volumes of information and shifting their attention from one topic to another. In particular, the evidence suggests that people can only hold a few pieces of information in their "working memory"—the brain system that maintains and manipulates information for several seconds during the planning and execution of many cognitive tasks[177] – at any given time.[178] These inherent human limitations will present an issue in a new health care system that is characterized by large volumes of data collection and dissemination. As noted in previous chapters in this volume, there are existing and emerging technologies, such as artificial intelligence and machine learning, that have the potential to sort, analyze, and send information to those who are best positioned to act on it. However, a number of questions will first need to be answered in order to build an effective system, including the following:

- Where will data be sent and stored? How will the data be protected?

- How will a given health care system, or the actors within it, decide if the data reveal a problem that needs to be addressed? What will the individuals or system do when there is a lack of data, for example, if a patient goes several days without using a remote monitoring system that is meant to collect data daily?

- What are the "trigger points" at which the system will notify someone regarding a problem?

- Who will the system notify? The patient, the provider, or someone else?

- How will the system notify a person, and how will the notification vary depending on the urgency of the situation? For example, notifications could range from text messages to patients to calling emergency services.

In short, the system must be built in order to *get the right information to the right person at the right time.* In addition, any system must be built with an eye toward the future, and must be able to contend with future technologies and the ever-growing number and complexity of data. Other issues will arise around sharing of these data, and maintaining data privacy and security, as discussed at great length in the regulatory chapter of this volume.

Issues Affecting Patients

Aside from the general issues that would govern all users of technology in a more distributed health care system, work stream participants cited a number of concerns specific to individuals and patients. These include the usability and accessibility of technologies to all people, regardless of cognitive or physical ability or geographic location; the potential difficulties of self-administering and self-monitoring various medical apparatuses; the fact that different patients are likely to have different ideas about how much and what kinds of technology they want to use; and the potential for new technologies to cause or exacerbate social isolation.

Accessibility

Making technology accessible to all people requires thinking through a variety of issues that may affect their abilities to use new technologies. The work stream cited key issues that must be considered: ensuring that technologies are accessible to people with all abilities, including people with low health literacy, low technological literacy, impaired hearing or sight, and physical and cognitive impairment; ensuring that a diverse group of stakeholders are involved in creating and implementing new technologies; exploring how generational, ethnic, racial, and other differences among people will impact the use of technology use; and addressing the issue of who will step in to assist patients, and how, when the technology doesn't work (an issue also addressed by the Work Force Work Stream in the previous chapter).

Technologies need to be developed in such a way that they are appropriate for people of all abilities. Technology developers should take this reality into account, and develop technologies that are usable for people with poor eyesight or hearing, appropriate for those with cognitive issues, and easy for all people to set up and use. Implementation of technologies also requires considering these factors. For example, technology should be introduced early in cases where the patient's cognition or eyesight are declining, so that the patient becomes comfortable with it. Incorporating new forms of voice-enabled technology—such as Amazon's Alexa, Apple's Siri, or Google's Assistant—may be the best way to ensure that technologies are easy to use for most people, regardless of their literacy or comfort with technology. However, there is limited evidence at this point about how well these voice-enabled systems will work for people with particular conditions, such as dementia.

Technologies should also be developed and implemented in a way that considers the fact that not all people have access to high-speed internet and up-to-date devices. For example, people who live in rural areas may not have cell phone or internet service that is adequate to access and use web-based tools, as discussed in Chapter III. Many low-literacy populations also sometimes lack good internet access, and many can only access the internet via a smartphone, but electronic health records and other information are at present typically designed to be viewed on a computer rather than a mobile phone (although mobile apps to EHRs are evolving). Tools and technologies for health care should be designed in such a way that they can be accessed on a variety of internet-capable systems.

To make care accessible to all, patients who lack the ability to view their health record online or interact with their provider via a health portal could benefit from a care coordinator, navigator, or community health worker, as discussed more fully in the work force chapter of this volume. This could be a person with less advanced training (i.e. not a clinician), who could be available by phone to go over the patient's medical record, their recorded interactions with their providers, and their provider's advice, and answer any questions that the patient may have. Although low-literacy patients would particularly benefit from such a program, it could be useful for all patients, given that nearly everyone has low health literacy at times—for example, when just receiving a devastating or particularly complex diagnosis.

Another fairly simple use of technology that has the potential to benefit many patients, caretakers, and families is recording provider-patient interactions. It has been demonstrated that patients retain very little of what their providers tell them,[179] so recording interactions would be enormously helpful, particularly for patients with low literacy or cognitive impairments. This use of technology could also be helpful for involving family and other caretakers. Those who can't participate in doctor appointments in-person could catch up later by watching the recording, and could help patients remember and understand the conversation.

Many of the populations who have the biggest barriers to using technologies—for example, people living in rural areas or low-literacy patients – are also those who might benefit the most. The challenge moving forward is to find a way to develop and implement technology in such a way that it is accessible and easy-to-use for all patients.

Self-Administration and Self Care

Because many of the emerging technologies will be used outside of the walls of traditional health care, patients will need to be able to activate and manage the technologies with minimal assistance. Some technologies may require little to no input from the patient: For example, a patient living alone could benefit from embedded machine vision technologies that could detect whether the patient is moving around the home and whether there are significant changes in gait that may indicate a problem, technologies that could indicate whether the patient has opened the refrigerator to eat something, and devices that could prompt the patient to take her medicine or perform other self-care.

At the other extreme are technologies that will require a greater level of effort and understanding from the patient, and probably at least some external assistance to ensure that the technologies work. Consider a patient who is prescribed a connected cuff to record blood pressure, along with a few wellness apps to manage exercise and diet. First, the patient may have to download the apps and sign up for their related services, which could require the ability to vet the user agreements of each of the technology providers. Next, the patient might have to figure out how to use the technology—for example, linking the blood pressure cuff with one's cellphone. As discussed in the work force chapter, a type of health technology assistant could support the patient in setting up the prescribed technologies, and may be needed to troubleshoot problems that could arise with a patient's home internet connection.

Similarly, a home-based ultrasound machine may have benefits for a patient who cannot travel to a traditional health clinic, but the benefits might not exceed the dangers of the patient using the machine incorrectly. There is the possibility that user error could result in the machine not detecting the fetus's heartbeat, and this error could result in emotional turmoil as well as a cascade of unnecessary and costly interventions. In order to prevent this type of problem, complex home-based technologies could be offered in concert with clinical and technological support via phone or internet, or community clinics such as CVS MinuteClinics could help bridge the gap between home technology and the clinic.

Patient Choice and Education

People have different views of technologies, and different ideas of how much technology is appropriate in their health care and their homes. When developing and implementing new technologies, it will be critical for leaders to keep in mind these differences. Patients should be able to choose the level and types of technology that are involved in their care, and health systems should ensure that patients who do not want certain technologies are not left behind.

For example, some patients may be quite happy to have a robot in their home that interacts with the patient and helps providers keep track of biometrics and wellbeing, while other patients may be uneasy with a robot and uninterested in these benefits. Some patients may enjoy using wearable technologies and be interested in looking at the data that are generated, while other patients may want little or nothing to do with these devices.

These differences in patient preferences may present a challenge for providers and care coordinators. If a health care system is set up with the assumption that patients will use email to contact their provider between appointments, how will the system ensure that a patient who cannot or will not use email is still able to contact their provider if needed?

The desire to use technology may also differ between patients and their personal care givers. For example, an in-home robot that monitors an elderly person and detects problems may be a welcome relief to a care giver, but the elderly person himself or herself may be reluctant to use it. Some of these divisions may fade as over time given younger individuals' general degree of comfort with technology. However, as long as some patients have different preferences about technology, it is critical that the health care or long-term care system account for these differences and provide equal access to care for all patients.

Aside from specific patient preferences regarding technology, there are also situations or diagnoses that may be more or less appropriate for the use of technology. Some patients with mental or behavioral health issues may benefit from online therapy; others may prefer being in the physical presence of a clinician. Educating patients about choices so that they can make informed decisions about which if any technologies they want to incorporate into their care will be important. Few providers are likely to know all the details about each technology that is available, and technologies are constantly changing. A system needs to be in place in order to ensure that patients know all their available options, can make informed choices, and can understand how these choices will impact their quality of life.

Social Isolation and Social Implications

A broad concern with all new technologies—not just health care technologies—is the potential that they will cause social isolation or have other wide-ranging social implications. The work stream stressed that the development and implementation of technology should be done in a way that facilitates and enriches human interaction, rather than replacing or weakening these relationships.

The concern about exacerbating social isolation and loneliness springs in part from a growing body of evidence demonstrating the ill effect of these conditions on health, particularly for older individuals. It is estimated that more than 8 million adults over age 50 in the United States are affected by isolation.[180] At least one study has found that for adults over age 60, loneliness was a predictor of functional decline and death. Adults who considered themselves lonely were more likely to experience declines in the activities of daily living and in mobility. Loneliness was also associated with an increased risk of death from such conditions as chronic hypertension and inflammation.[181]

New technology, of course, has the potential both to exacerbate isolation and loneliness or to mitigate it. If avatars or robots are used to replace human interaction—for example, in-home robots rather than in-home human caretakers—there is the potential for people to become isolated from their family, friends, and communities. There has been little research to date on this issue, however, and it will need to be studied thoroughly as technologies come into broader use.

At the same time, it is clearly the case that technology need not completely replace physical human-to-human interactions, but can instead augment or facilitate less direct forms of interactions to address care needs. For example, CareCoach, a digital eldercare service, employs avatars featured on tablets that are actually directed by human care coaches who observe those in need of care remotely. For about $200 a month, the system can watch over a homebound person around the clock, and keep family members or other remote caregivers fully informed about the person's situation. In one case, recounted in a story in Wired, an elderly man became so personally connected to the avatar, a cartoon dog, that his daughter brought the tablet featuring the avatar along to the man's funeral after he eventually died.[182]

Robots in particular are likely to become a valuable adjunct to provision of in-person or remote care. A robot in the home of an elderly person could order a Lyft or Uber to take the person to coffee with friends, or could alert a friend or family member if the person was having problems or wasn't responding. A wide array of robots already in use in some eldercare facilities in Japan are used to help caregivers get patients out of bed or transfer to wheelchairs; some even mimic live therapy animals.[183] In addition to relieving some of the physical burdens of providing care, robots can relieve some of the emotional burden of caregiving. A person with dementia can ask a robot twenty times in a row what time it is, and the robot will never become frustrated or upset—in effect, providing a small amount of at least temporary respite for an actual human caregiver.

Technology can also be a means of increasing social support in the virtual world. Patients can be connected with online group therapy sessions or peer support groups for specific diseases or conditions. Social media portals for patients with the same condition could implement approaches such as so-called voluntary indicators of health. For example, if a patient's blood sugar has been kept under control for a certain amount of time, he or she would get a green badge visible to other members of the social group. This approach could be particularly helpful for patients who are less able to connect with peers in person due to issues such as geographic isolation, rare diseases, or physical or psychological conditions that impede being physically present at a meeting.

Issues Affecting Providers

With the introduction of new technologies into the health care system, the respective roles and responsibilities of providers and patients are likely to change. For technologies to be successfully implemented in the day-to-day practice of health care, it will be essential for providers to understand and trust them, and to accept and accommodate the corresponding role changes. Otherwise, if clinicians are resistant to, or anxious about, such steps as making medical decisions through the use of technology (e.g. telemedicine visits), patients may pick up on their providers' anxiety and lose confidence in the system and in the medical decisions being made.

Relatively little is known about health professionals' attitudes toward the use of new technologies in health care. However, broadly speaking, as providers gain more experience with new technologies, their attitudes may shift. Some recent technological advances—such as electronic health records—have been seen by providers as further burdening their workload. However, some of the technologies of the future have the potential to help providers better serve their patients and to lighten their workload. For example, while providers may be expected to monitor and assess a deluge of data points, they may also be able to share some aspects of their workload with intelligent agents and computerized clinical decision support tools. These benefits to providers may reduce resistance to new technologies, although this issue, too, will need to be studied over time.

In addition to relieving the workload of individual providers, technology has the potential to reduce the costs and increase the efficiencies of the health care system as a whole. Health care is an extremely labor-intensive industry, and labor costs constitute the largest single source of costs in health care systems. As noted in the work force chapter of this volume, reducing overall health care costs, while also expanding access, will require achieving greater labor efficiencies. Because demand for health care is to some degree unlimited—and because supply of clinicians can often create its own demand—perceived shortages of clinicians in some sense will never abate. Delivering health care efficiently will require reducing the labor intensity of health care, not adding more personnel or labor inputs or adding more duties to a providers' plate.

In a more distributed, digitally-enabled system, there will be multiple opportunities for "task-shifting," a strategy commonly used in health systems in low resource countries and settings, but less commonly used in the United States.[184] The current health care system—particularly mental health care—is very clinician-dependent and relies on clinicians to do much of the heavy lifting. However, systems in countries such as China use their clinicians at "higher" levels of health care, with workers who have less education and training doing much of the frontline work. Technology may enable the U.S. system to similarly leverage the unique skills and knowledge of clinicians while using technologies such as AI, avatars, or decision support to help with provision of frontline care. These advances in technology may make it possible for health care to be provided to everyone in need, by reducing inefficiencies and freeing up providers so that they can focus on patient care.

As also addressed in the work force chapter, successful implementation of new technologies in health care will require careful thought about work flow, and potentially substantial redesign of it. At the same time, new technologies will have to take account of the ways that providers are accustomed to practicing medicine. For example, providers traditionally use their bodies and their senses to practice medicine and to make decisions. Physicians assess a patient's heartbeat through their own body's senses of hearing and feeling, and while some technology has the capacity to enhance these assessments (e.g. a remote stethoscope that can amplify and record the heartbeat), other technologies may hinder a provider's ability to assess a patient (e.g. a telehealth visit does not allow the provider to use the sense of touch).

Recommendations

The Human Factors Work Stream issued recommendations falling into several categories, as set forth below. An initial set of general recommendations is aimed at the large overall group of stakeholders, including technology developers and health care organizations. Recommendations directed to those specific groups, along with institutions of health professions education and training, and regulators, follow.

GENERAL RECOMMENDATIONS

As already discussed in this chapter, most technology developers understand and take into account human factors when creating new technologies, and health systems have also benefited from taking human factors into account when they adopt computerized physician order entry and other health information technology systems.[185] It will be especially important that technology developers and adopters take these factors into account as they devise and adopt technologies to be used in distributed health care settings. They, along with the health care organizations and others that take up and deploy these technologies, will need to understand the convergence of technology with human factors such as physical or mental abilities, cultural and generational differences, comfort with and aptitude to use technology, and the physical environment in which the technology will be used.

If technology developers do not consider the convergence of the technology and the user, the technology is unlikely to be adopted, or if adopted, used effectively and appropriately. Technology developers along with health care organizations have an obligation to get new technologies "right" when it comes not just to important factors such as safety, efficacy, and affordability, but also to factors such as usability and appropriate tailoring of the technology to the specific human context in which it will be used.

As a result, it would be most desirable to have a set of overarching principles and easy-to-use methods of human-centered design specifically to be applied to development of health-care related technologies. These principles could be incorporated into a set of voluntary standards that both developers and users of these technologies would endorse and abide by. To the maximum degree possible, these principles should be based on evidence; technology developers should be able to see direct linkages between these principles and the ultimate success of their products in the marketplace, and thus, to a return on investment.

These principles and voluntary standards are likely to be most useful if they describe desirable processes for incorporating human factors into product design and development, as well as achieving overall outcomes. For example, standards could describe how technology developers would meaningfully go about determining the usability of their products and appropriateness for specific types of users, rather than determining product specifications – e.g., font size of type appearing on a screen. Technologies can then be tested in studies to document whether or not they achieve the intended results.

To derive such a voluntary set of standards, the American Hospital Association, the American Medical Association, the American Nursing Association or other credible health care organization could join with a technology industry group, and with organizations such as the Human Factors and Ergonomics Society, the Usability Professionals Association, the Association for Computing Machinery, and SIG-CHI (the Special Interest Group on Computer-Human Interaction). In turn, these combined organizations could convene a broad group of stakeholders – technology developers, health systems, human factors professionals, health clinicians, and representatives of patient and consumer groups – to frame the most critical human factors considerations and propose processes for addressing them that could be incorporated into the industry standard. Much as safer-to-use needles aimed at minimizing or preventing accidental needlesticks of health care workers were developed by industry working in collaboration with clinicians and design professionals, working collaboratives could also be devised to address usability and human factors issues that arise as the development of new technologies continues.

To Technology Developers

There are several approaches that developers could take on their own to expand the consideration of human factors in their work, as follows:

1. Technology developers should be educated about human factors, either in the formal educational setting, in the course of business, or in ongoing professional development.

2. Technology developers should increase the diversity of the technology development work force. Having a more diverse work force will best equip developers to produce technology that is more likely to be usable by, and attractive to, different types of users. As Microsoft CEO Satya Nadella has put it, "Inclusive teams that value diverse perspectives and inclusive design principles will have the deepest impact in building products designed for everyone."

3. Technology developers should utilize co-creation approaches, in which end users (e.g. clinicians and other health care workers, and patients or consumers) are involved in the development of technology from the earliest stages. Technology developers should consider having advisory boards that focus on such issues as diversity and usability and have meaningful input into the design and development of technologies.

To Health Care Organizations

Health care organizations need to integrate human factors expertise into many facets of health care delivery, and should incorporate the input of human factors experts into such areas as provider education, simulation, quality improvement, patient experience, and procurement. Specifically:

1. Health care organizations should proactively engage with technology developers to create usable, useful, and safe technologies, and should not wait until technology developers come to them.

2. Health care organizations' decisions to purchase or procure technologies should be made with the input of a multidisciplinary, patient-focused team that includes human factors experts, health professionals of all types, and patients. Patient advisory councils may be especially useful when vetting new technologies or practices.

3. Health care organizations need to be aware and sensitive to the different needs and wants of patients, and not assume that one size fits all. Different models of care may be appropriate for different patients, and the use of technology may be appropriate at certain stages but not others. Technology should be used to improve the human connection between a patient and provider, rather than to replace it.

4. Health care organizations should regularly perform "ride alongs" in order to understand the patient experience. In a ride along, someone acts as a patient (e.g. lives in a senior facility for a month) in order to observe and document what the experience is like for the patient, so that the health care organization can devise appropriate processes and best ways of employing technologies.

To Institutions of Health Education and Training

In light of advances in technology and its growing use in health care, health professions education should be restructured, as recommended in the previous Work Force chapter. As health professions education and training incorporates instruction on the provision of virtual care, it should also provide at least some amount of training in human factors and human-centered design, either as part of a degree curriculum or as continuing education. Simulations in particular can be used in pursuit of a number of learning objectives, including the acquisition of technical skills, learning new processes, or improving team work.

To Regulators and Government Agencies

1. In the case of technologies that are subject to regulatory approvals, either by the Food and Drug Administration or other regulatory agencies, the regulatory system should employ some mix of carrot-and-stick approaches

to encourage consideration of human factors in the development and adoption of technologies. Carrots, or incentives, should be tried first, to be followed by sticks, or penalties, if these do not work.

2. In the "carrot" approach, the consideration of usability and human factors would be encouraged through the promise of faster or easier product approval for organizations participating in such programs. The Centers for Medicare and Medicaid Services (CMS), as well as the Center for Medicare and Medicaid Innovation (CMMI), could also speed approvals of demonstration projects or other tests that incorporated human-centered design into any technological applications that are part of an innovative payment or delivery reform initiative.

3. In a "stick" approach, regulators could enforce the consideration of usability and human factors issues through the regulatory process. For example, regulators such as FDA could require that tech developers involve end users in the design process. Much as the 21st Century Cures Act emphasized the need for patient engagement in the development of new biopharmaceuticals, a new law or regulations could encourage or require patient input into technology development.

4. In the pre-certification program now being piloted by FDA (see regulatory chapter for further discussion), the involvement of end users in design of a product or technology should be a criterion of qualification for a company to participate.

5. A voluntary industry standard should be adopted, as described above, that requires involving patients in product design; or a voluntary system of ranking or a seal of "approval" from the National Institute for Standards and Technology or other entity for technologies should be awarded to technologies that are developed with usability and human factors in mind.

Knowledge Gaps

The future development and adoption of health-care related technologies will pose potentially countless research questions bearing on human factors issues. Rather than specify a list of research topics, the Human Factors Work Stream chose to spell out key areas of research that will be needed to fill knowledge gaps.

1. **Usability and safety:** What are key features of new technologies that make them generally more useful, and safer, and more likely to be adopted?

2. **Contribution to social isolation**: As noted previously in this chapter, there is some concern that new technology has the potential on the one hand to exacerbate isolation, and on the other hand, to mitigate it. There has been little research to date on this issue, however, and it will need to be studied thoroughly as technologies come into broader use.

3. **Incorporation into work flow:** What features of new technologies have the greatest potential to help providers better serve their patients, lighten their workload, and minimize clinician "burnout?"

4. **Processing of data and information**: What features of new technologies, or systems, will best enable both patients and providers to meaningfully assess and act on the volumes of data and information that will be collected through remote monitoring and other technologies?

5. **Limits on use:** What if any are appropriate limits on the use of virtual technologies in health care? Should best practices be promulgated that contain "trigger points" for health systems and others to decide when virtual technologies are appropriate. For example, can or should important discussions about end-of-life care be had virtually, such as via telehealth? Should a person be informed in a telehealth "visit" that he or she has dementia? Should an avatar enabled by artificial intelligence hold an end-of-life "discussion" with a patient? These are not just research but also ethical questions that should be surfaced and explored.

Conclusion

Technologies that enable and support the ability of more health care to be delivered virtually when appropriate, or to move closer to individuals in their homes and communities, are already in use, and are likely to be even more so in the future. To realize the utmost potential of care delivered with the aid of these technologies, they must be developed and adopted in ways that take into account interactions between humans and technologies; the rest of the sociotechnical system (e.g., the physical and social environment in which technologies will be used); and the attitudes, biases, and beliefs that may affect how patients and providers view and use technologies.

Technologies useful in health care should be viewed as a means of enabling different forms of human interactions around the care process, rather than always replacing those interactions. Technology developers—and those who deploy and use technologies in the health care system—must acknowledge and address the different preferences and abilities of humans to use technologies appropriately. Providers and patients will experience growing pains as they shift into new roles and take on new responsibilities, and the health care education system as well as health system leaders will need to prepare the work force for these changes. There are many likely upsides to a more distributed health care system, but these advances are only possible if the multiple human factors discussed in this white paper are considered, and dealt with, in the design and deployment of technologies within the evolving system.

Human Factors in Designing Heath Care Without Walls: Chapter 5 in Brief

1. The profound changes that are occurring in how health care services and supports are delivered, with care moving out of conventional health care settings thanks to technologies such as telehealth and remote monitoring, will cause further sweeping changes in the ways that individuals and health care professionals engage with each other—not just for given care episodes, but over their lifetimes. Some technologies will also be used to displace humans and actually provide care to patients—for example, by robots. Health-related technologies may also surround humans in their everyday environments—for example, to monitor individuals' biometric data; and feed the information back into patients' electronic health records or applications.

2. As Health Care Without Walls unfolds, it is critical that attention be paid not just to the technologies themselves, but to the human factors that will determine how successfully and to what extent these technologies are integrated into health care. The field of human factors is the scientific discipline concerned with the understanding of interactions among humans and other elements of a system, and with applying what is known about humans' behavior, abilities, limitations, and other characteristics to the design of systems, activities, environments, and equipment or technologies. Human factors, for example, might be invoked to understand why people will react differently to a robot that features a human-like face versus one that resembles a mere machine.

3. The Human Factors Work Stream of the Health Care Without Walls initiative thus sought to delineate the relevant issues that technology developers, health systems, educational and training systems and others should address in order to facilitate the evolution of a patient-centric, distributed health care system. It also recommended changes in public policy, and within health systems and other organizations, to support the 2025 Health Care Without Walls vision.

4. The work stream concluded that emerging technologies used in health care must be considered as part of the broader "sociotechnical" system, in which technologies interact with the social and physical realities of the world and with people's beliefs and abilities. Understanding the sociotechnical system requires a multidisciplinary view, using approaches including human factors and ergonomics, behavioral economics, sociology, psychology, and human-centered design. Exploring new technologies through this broad, multidisciplinary perspective is essential in order to fully understand the promises and pitfalls of a new world of "Health Care Without Walls."

5. Such a multidisciplinary perspective suggests that, if new technologies are to be used effectively in health care, they should be based on a number of core principles. Among them: Technologies should be created through human-centered design—a process that starts with people and ends with solutions tailored to suit their needs. Technologies should be easy to use and "frictionless" for different types of users with different abilities, and seamlessly integrated into their lives so that they become an almost invisible part of the health care journey. Technologies should be predicated on the seamless ability to exchange data within appropriate security and privacy safeguards; to allow data to follow patients; and to present data in such a way that they are clearly understood and actionable for users. They should not only be safe when used correctly, but should also incorporate fail-safe mechanisms and backstops that will prevent injury or death in the event that they are not used correctly.

6. The core principles described above should be incorporated into a set of voluntary standards that both developers and users of these technologies would endorse and abide by. To derive such standards, organizations such as the American Hospital Association, the American Medical Association, the American Nursing Association and others could join with a technology

industry group, and with organizations such as the Human Factors and Ergonomics Society, to convene stakeholders and to frame standards.

7. Technology developers should take steps on their own to expand their consideration and application of human factors. For example, having a more diverse work force will best equip developers to produce technology that is more likely to be usable by, and attractive to, different types of users. A voluntary industry standard also should be adopted that requires involving patients in product design; or a voluntary system of ranking or a seal of "approval" created for technologies that are developed with usability and human factors in mind.

8. In the case of technologies that are subject to regulatory approvals, either by the Food and Drug Administration or other regulatory agencies, the regulatory system should employ some mix of carrot-and-stick approaches to encourage consideration of human factors in the development and adoption of technologies. In the "carrot" approach, the consideration of usability and human factors would be encouraged through the promise of faster or easier product approval for organizations participating in such programs. In a "stick" approach, regulators could enforce the consideration of usability and human factors issues through the regulatory process. For example, in the pre-certification program now being piloted by FDA, the involvement of end users in design of a product or technology should be a criterion of qualification for a company to participate. In general, carrots, or incentives, should be tried first, to be followed by sticks, or penalties, if these do not work.

9. Health care organizations should integrate human factors expertise into many facets of health care delivery, including virtual care, and should incorporate the input of human factors experts into such areas as provider education, simulation, quality improvement, evaluation of patient experience, and technology procurement. An example would be conducting "ride alongs," in which someone acts as a patient in order to observe and document what the experience of using a particular technology is like for the patient. Health care organizations also should proactively engage with technology developers to create usable, useful, and safe technologies, and should not wait until technology developers come to them.

10. As health professions education and training is restructured to incorporate instruction in virtual care, it should require at least some amount of training

in human factors and human-centered design, either as part of a degree curriculum or as continuing education.

11. Multiple knowledge gaps exist, and both the public and private sectors should invest in research that will shed light on human factors considerations as Health Care Without Walls evolves. Especially important will be identifying key features of technologies that make them generally more useful, and safer, and more likely to be adopted by health care providers and patients alike. Other key questions include whether use of more virtual technologies in health care will exacerbate isolation, or mitigate it; what features of new technologies have the greatest potential to help providers better serve their patients, lighten their workload, and minimize clinician "burnout;" and what if any are appropriate limits on the use of virtual technologies in health care, such as in discussions about end-of-life care. Some of these topics may not just amount to research questions, but also ethical ones to be explored.

◆ ◆ ◆

End Notes, Chapter 5

[149] See https://www.iea.cc/whats.

[150] National Research Council, *Health Care Comes Home: The Human Factors* (Washington, DC: The National Academies Press, 2011), 61.

[151] Susanne Buck, "Nine human factors contributing to the user acceptance of telemedicine applications: a cognitive-emotional approach," *Journal of Telemedicine and Telecare* 15, no.2(March 2009):55-8, DOI: 10.1258/jtt.2008.008007.

[152] Pascale Carayon, "Human factors of complex sociotechnical systems," *Applied ergonomics* 37, no.4(2006):525-535, https://doi.org/10.1016/j.apergo.2006.04.011.

[153] Pascale Carayon et al., "Work system design for patient safety: the SEIPS model," *BMJ Quality & Safety* 15, no. suppl 1(2006):i50-i58, DOI: 10.1136/qshc.2005.015842.

[154] See http://www.designkit.org/human-centered-design.

[155] Emily Singer, "The Virtual Nurse Will See You Now," MIT Technology Review, November 1, 2011, https://www.technologyreview.com/s/425983/the-virtual-nurse-will-see-you-now/.

[156] Frances Dare, "Can High Tech Be High Touch in Healthcare?," Accenture, May 3, 2017, https://www.accenture.com/us-en/blogs/blogs-high-tech-high-touch-healthcare.

[157] Dominic Howell, "Virtual therapy 'helps with depression', researchers say," BBC News, February 15, 2016, http://www.bbc.com/news/uk-35558447.

[158] Jennifer Kite-Powell, "Using Virtual And Augmented Reality In Medical Diagnosis, Treatment and Therapy," Forbes, September 30, 2017,

https://www.forbes.com/sites/jenniferhicks/2017/09/20/using-virtual-and-augmented-reality-in-medical-diagnosis-treatment-and-therapy/#686b674fc4bc.

[159] See https://www.england.nhs.uk/wp-content/uploads/2014/12/tecs-flo.pdf.

[160] "33,000 patients go with the Flo," digitalhealth, February 12, 2016, https://www.digitalhealth.net/2016/02/33000-patients-go-with-the-flo/.

[161] Jenny Deam, "Live-stream app helps families connect with NICU babies," Houston Chronicle, October 20, 2017, https://www.houstonchronicle.com/business/medical/article/Live-stream-app-helps-families-connect-with-NICU-12294449.php.

[162] Mitchell Northam, "Parents can now watch live video of NICU babies at N. Fulton hospital," The Atlanta Journal-Constitution, September 07, 2017, https://www.ajc.com/news/local/parents-can-now-watch-live-video-nicu-babies-fulton-hospital/0jwZZlQEDPBkRUmIhsPhpO/.

[163] See https://www.bigwhitewall.com/home/how-it-works.aspx#.Wz5ozNVKipo.

[164] See https://www.silvercloudhealth.com/us/blog/article/gallagher-student-health-partners-with-silvercloud-health-to-bring-behavior.

[165] See https://golantern.com/.

[166] Paul Fronstin and Edna Dretzka, "Consumer Engagement in Health Care Among Millennials, Baby Boomers, and Generation X: Findings from the 2017 Consumer Engagement in Health Care Survey," Employee Benefit Research Institute, March 5, 2018, https://www.ebri.org/pdf/briefspdf/EBRI_IB_444.pdf.

[167] Karen Adams, Ann C. Greiner, and Janet M. Corrigan, Committee on the Crossing the Quality Chasm: Next Steps Toward a New Health Care System. *The 1st Annual Crossing the Quality Chasm Summit: A Focus on Communities.* (Washington, DC: National Academies Press, 2004).

[168] Robert S Rudin and David W Bates, "Let the left hand know what the right is doing: A vision for care coordination and electronic health records," *Journal of the American Medical Informatics Association* 21, no. 1. (January 2014): 13-16, DOI: 10.1136/amiajnl-2013-001737.

[169] Raja Parasuraman, Thomas B. Sheridan and Christopher D. Wickens, "A model for types and levels of human interaction with automation," *IEEE Transactions on systems, man, and cybernetics-Part A: Systems and Humans* 30, no. 3 (2000): 286-297.

[170] See https://www.uaspire.org/.

[171] See https://www.text4baby.org/.

[172] Eric J. Topol, *The patient will see you now: the future of medicine is in your hands*, (Tantor Media, 2015).

[173] Irma Klerings, Alexandra S. Weindhandl, and Kylie J. Thaler, "Information overload in healthcare: too much of a good thing?" *Zeitschrift für Evidenz, Fortbildung und Qualität im Gesundheitswesen* 109, no.4-5 (2015):289-290. DOI:10.1016/j.zefq.2015.06.005.

[174] Katherine G. Footracer, "Alert fatigue in electronic health records," *Journal of the American Academy of PAs* 28, no. 7(July 2015):41-42, DOI:10.1097/01.JAA.0000465221.04234.ca.

[175] Eyal Ophir, Clifford Nass, and Anthony D. Wagner, "Cognitive control in media multitaskers," *Proceedings of the National Academy of Sciences* 106, no. 37(2009):15583-15587, https://doi.org/10.1073/pnas.0903620106.

[176] Mona Moisala et al., "Media multitasking is associated with distractibility and increased prefrontal activity in adolescents and young adults," *NeuroImage* 134, (July 2016): 113-121, https://doi.org/10.1016/j.neuroimage.2016.04.011.

[177] Omri Barak and Misha Tsodyks, "Working models of working memory," *Current opinion in neurobiology* 25, (April 2014):20-24, DOI:10.1016/j.conb.2013.10.008.

[178] Nelson Cowan, "The magical number 4 in short-term memory: a reconsideration of mental storage capacity," *Behavioral and Brain Sciences* 24, no.1(February 2001):87-114.

[179] Paula Span, "The Appointment Ends. Now the Patient is Listening." New York Times, August 18, 2017, https://www.nytimes.com/2017/08/18/health/recording-your-doctors-appointment.html.

[180] See "Connect2Affect," the AARP Foundation, at https://connect2affect.org/about-isolation/.

[181] Carla M. Perissinotto, Irena Stijacic Cenzer, and Kenneth E. Covinsky, "Loneliness in older persons: a predictor of functional decline and death," *Archives of internal medicine* 172, no.14 (2012):1078-1084, DOI:10.1001/archinternmed.2012.1993.

[182] Lauren Smiley, "What happens when we let tech care for our aging parents," The Wired, December 19, 2017, https://www.wired.com/story/digital-puppy-seniors-nursing-homes/.

[183] Malcolm Foster, "Ageing Japan: Robots may have role in future of elder care," AOL, March 27, 2018, https://www.aol.com/article/news/2018/03/27/ageing-japan-robots-may-have-role-in-future-of-elder-care/23397072/.

[184] See *"Task Shifting Global Recommendations and Guidelines,"* World Health Organization, 2007, http://www.unaids.org/sites/default/files/media_asset/ttr_taskshifting_en_0.pdf.

[185] For example, see Ann Schoofs Hundt et al., "Conducting an efficient proactive risk assessment prior to CPOE implementation," *International Journal of Medical Informatics* 82, no. 1(2013): 25-38, DOI: 10.1016/j.ijmedinf.2012.04.005; also see Ann Schoofs Hundt, "A collaborative usability evaluation (CUE) model for health IT design and implementation," *International Journal of Human-Computer Interaction* 33, no. 4: 287-297, https://doi.org/10.1080/10447318.2016.1263430.

SCENARIO 8: VIRTUAL CARE AND PANDEMIC INFLUENZA

IT'S LATE SUMMER in the United States, a couple of months before the onset of flu season, when news reports from Australia and China tell of an apparently new strain of virus that has all the hallmarks of being a pandemic. As the virus spreads to parts of the Far East, death rates are high, especially among younger people. Shipments of annual flu vaccine, engineered for other flu strains, are already under way in the United States. However, in September and October, hot spots of this new flu strain begin to appear in a few major U.S. cities.

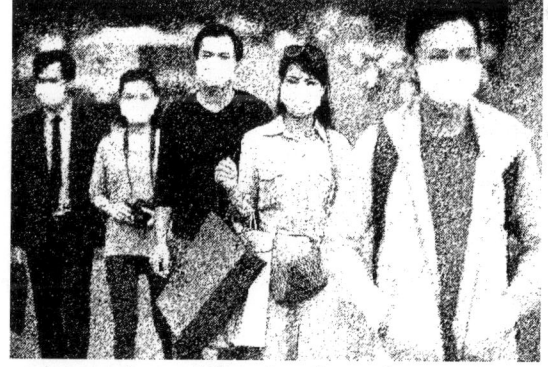

Federal and state public health officials step in and begin instituting various measures, including quarantining those believed to have been exposed to the new flu virus, isolating those who are sick, and undertaking various social distancing measures, such as school closings. Suddenly, local health systems in many jurisdictions are overrun with sick patients, while public health authorities must deal with panic in some quarters and the after-effects of social isolation measures, including anxiety and depression.

In a typical year, approximately 5 percent to 20 percent of the U.S. population will become ill each year with seasonal influenza; approximately 200,000 will be hospitalized, anywhere from 3,000 to 49,000 will die. Overall, influenzas and pneumonia were the 8th leading cause of death in 2014. However, an influenza pandemic occurs when a new influenza virus emerges and spreads around the world, often before an effective vaccine is developed. The most recent influenza pandemic began in 2009, when a novel influenza A type, H1N1, colloquially known as "swine flu," emerged. From April 2009 to April 2010, the Centers for Disease Control and Prevention estimated that there were 60.8 million cases in the United States and nearly 12,500 deaths.

In the event of a flu pandemic, millions would need to be monitored for flu symptoms, and if infection is suspected or evident, treated with antivirals and other medications. Additional strategies that have been developed for dealing with pandemic influenza include quarantine (separating and restricting the movement of people exposed to a contagious disease); isolation (separating sick people from those who are not sick), and social distancing (various actions taken by public health authorities to control the spread of contagious illnesses including school and workplace closures, cancellation of mass gatherings, shutting down or limiting mass transit, among others).

What could "Health Care Without Walls" approaches look like in the event of a flu pandemic?

Symptom monitoring: Digital thermometers, as well as wireless thermometer devices linked to smart phones, could be broadly distributed by public health authorities. In the past, some airports around the world have deployed thermal imaging cameras to see whether travelers have fevers; these could also be deployed in locations in major cities. There could also be mass distribution of influenza rapid diagnostic tests (RIDTs), known as point-of- care tests (POCT) or 'dipsticks', that would detect specific influenza viral antigens or proteins in infected people. Information about positive tests could be directly transmitted to clinicians via photos snapped on smart phones or other methods.

Treating the sick: Caring for as many ill patients as possible in their homes with antivirals and other medications could be a vitally important strategy – both to prevent overcrowding of health systems, and also to minimize contagion. Telehealth visits with clinicians, triggered by positive flu tests, could help to firm up fly diagnoses. Uber and Lyft drivers, and/or fleets of autonomous cars, or even drones, could be dispatched to patient's homes or other locations to deliver antivirals and other medications. Pharmacy technicians, pharmaceutical delivery trucks, community health workers, and EMS response units could also be equipped to check in on and triage patients

For those who became seriously ill, hospital at home programs could be instituted, or drivers and autonomous cars dispatched to bring people to hospitals for care. Pop-up isolation units could be built and advanced, and distributed to hospitals and health units on an as-needed basis, to allow for onsite patient care.

Mass communications: Instructing people on symptom recognition, flu treatments, and the need for social isolation strategies would be critical. Emergency SMS text messaging systems could be used to inform people about the pandemic and what to do to obtain needed treatment. Psychologists, social workers and others could use telehealth to counsel individuals coping with quarantine or isolation, experiencing symptoms from social isolation, or they could conduct broad interventions to multiple individuals or larger populations with the assistance of apps. Federal, state, and local agencies would need to partner well in advance to plan for, purchase, equip, train, and carry out all of these interventions. Pilots of various approaches should be run in conventional flu seasons to test and refine approaches.

♦ ♦ ♦

Made in the USA
Middletown, DE
30 November 2018